Grigori Grabovoi

# Restoration of Matter of Human Being by Concentrating on Number Sequences

## Book 2

The work „Restoration of Matter of Human Being by Concentrating on Number Sequences" was created and supplemented by Grigori Grabovoi in 2002.

Hamburg

2013

Jelezky Publishing, Hamburg
www.jelezky-publishing.com

First English Edition, June 2013
© 2013 English Language Edition

Edition: 2013-1, 07.06.2013

SVET UG, Hamburg (Publisher)

Published by SVET UG, Hamburg, Germany 2013

For further information on the contents of this book contact:
SVET Centre, Hamburg

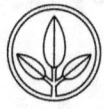

www.svet-centre.com

Copyright © 2013 SVET UG

The use of text and illustrations, also as excerpts, without the permission of the publisher is a violation of copyright law and punishable as such. This includes photocopies, translations, microfilm copies and data processing for electronic systems.

ISBN: 978-3-943110-75-3

© Грабовой Г.П. 2002

According to the responses we have received, the contents of this book have helped many people. We are confident that this will continue to be the case.

Nonetheless, we would like to point out that the techniques of Grigori Grabovoi are mental methods for the guidance of events in one's life. These methods are dependent upon one's personal spiritual development. Because we are dealing with topics relating to one's health, we give this express notice that such influence is not a "therapy" in the conventional sense of the word and is therefore not intended to limit or replace professional medical care.

When in doubt, follow the directions of your doctor or a therapist or pharmacist whom you trust!

(When following conventional methods, you must expect to get conventional results.)

Jelelezky Publishing/SVET Centre, Hamburg

Disclaimer:

The information within this book is intended as reference material only, and not as medical or professional advice.

Information contained herein is intended to give you the tools to make informed decisions about your lifestyle. It should not be used as a substitute for any treatment that has been prescribed or recommended by your qualified doctor. Do not stop taking any medication unless advised by your qualified doctor to do otherwise. The author and publisher are not healthcare professionals, and expressly disclaim any responsibility for any adverse effects occurring as a result of the use of suggestions or information in this book. This book is offered for your own education and enjoyment only. As always, never begin a health program without first consulting a qualified healthcare professional. Your use of this book indicates your agreement to these terms.

# INTRODUCTION

To restore the matter of human being with the numerical concentrations the following methods can be used:

1. Read the number sequence corresponding to matter being restored, written after the name of matter.

2. Pronounce mentally the number sequence corresponding to the matter being restored.

3. Look at the picture or the name of the matter being restored.

4. Imagine that you are situated between the numbers of the sequence, having big size, corresponding to the matter being recreated. You must strive to perceive clearly the numbers, between which you imagine yourself. The light of these numbers can reach you. These actions can be performed with any numbers of sequence.

5. Imagine that you are looking at the number sequence from above.

6. Imagine the number sequence in that area which you are restoring. To do this, you must use the image of the matter, given in this book, with the sequence of numbers you are using.

7. Imagine the number sequence between the picture of the matter and a part of the specular reflection, given in this book, which correspond to the

number sequence being used.

8. Comparing the numbers of the sequence, you can find a controlling relationship between the various kinds of human matter in the direction to norm. It is possible to restore the matter, using the number sequence corresponding to the other matter. At first you can concentrate on the numbers of the sequence of the other matter, which coincide with the numbers of the sequence of the matter being restored. Then you can use the whole sequence of numbers of the other matter, drawing in your thoughts a light beam which crosses the number sequence of the matter or the matter itself which you are restoring. At the perception of the rapid restoring effect you can define the next point or area in your body after the restored matter itself, through which the matter is recreated. This next point or area in such a case will be situated in the other matter, with the help of the number sequence of which the restoration of the matter, chosen by you, is carried out. There could be a lot of such following points or areas through which the creation of the matter is performed. The first point or area of the selected matter is in the matter itself.

Having found, through the use of number sequence, the points or areas of creation of the matter being restored, one can recreate the matter focusing his attention on these points or areas. At this time such a spiritual state sets in that corresponds to the restoration and the normal state of the chosen matter. Bringing back to memory and feeling again the same spiritual state, you can restore the matter by means of spirit, which thus is a Life-giving Spirit. Then you can extend this spiritual act to the whole matter of the body taking into account external events and thus achieve a spiritual state, corresponding to the eternal development.

In certain cases, depending on the angle of perception, different number sequences can correspond to the same matter being restored.

9. To accelerate the restoration of the human matter the gaps in the number sequences can be perceived as the gaps between the words in a sentence. Then for each component of a number sequence, separated by the gap, one can see a word that has a meaning of a normally functioning matter to which given number sequence corresponds. Then, trying to perceive this word, it is possible to perceive the Creator's level creating the matter that corresponds to the number sequence and the matter of the whole body. Light, creating the matter corresponding to the number sequence, is spread, according to the laws of optics, to all other matters of the human body and to the environment. From this you can understand why some feelings and emotions are perceived as external. This allows to recognize more accurately where on the level of control over events it is necessary to act on the basis of the interaction of body tissues and where on the basis of the interaction of the matter of the organism and the environment. This method of the exact detection allows you to make control over events more efficiently until the level of the normal state of matter of the body is reached, regardless of any circumstances.

With this method you perceive simultaneously both tissue of the body and the events surrounding a man in such a way as though you are looking at the described above with the physical eyes. And depending on situation, you can make a decision how to act in the direction of eternal development. In some cases you can perform physical actions, and in some periods you can perform a spiritual action for the normalization of the events in the direction to the eternal life.

Such perception of yours develops your spirit, soul and physical body to the level at which the creation of human matter is fulfilled on spiritual basis. Figures make it possible to get the exact spiritual state, corresponding to the norm of human matter. To strengthen the control you can use common known, that is well fixed in the collective consciousness, knowledge from physics, about the corpuscular-wave duality of matter, according to which any object can show both its wave properties and particle characteristics of matter. Creating the light waves by concentration on the number sequence corresponding to the normal human matter, you create normally functioning human matter.

All the methods of restoration of human matter with the help of concentration on number sequences given in this book can be used with preventive and sanitary purposes, for rejuvenation, and in case of necessity, to restore the matter, regardless of the initial data, on the basis of which the matter is restored. When using the described methods in paragraphs 1-9 in the introduction you can consider the following:

With the aim of prophylaxis it is expedient to make rehabilitation with the simultaneous spreading the effect of concentration on number sequences for the future.

For rejuvenation it is expedient to concentrate in succession at first on the number sequence, located in the content (of the book), taking into account the task of eternal development, and then concentrate on the matter which you are locally rejuvenating.

Restoring the matter of the body, you can perform concentration on number sequences in succession with the help of the various methods given in this book. You can use the number sequences corresponding to the matter being restored, as well as the number sequences of the area, which includes the matter you are restoring.

If it is necessary to restore the matter after biological death, then you should at first concentrate on the numbers consecutively from left to right, then in reverse order – from right to left.

The spiritual impulse creating human matter makes it possible to expand the methods of restoration. Restoring the human matter one must strive to develop the spiritual level to the state in which the matter is created and functions by the spiritual activity, along with the biological principles and principles of events. Such spiritual state in the process of implementation of the methods of the eternal development must ensure full restoration of human matter, regardless of the initial data and any circumstances.

© Грабовой Г.П. 2002

© Грабовой Г.П. 2002

# HEMOPOIETIC SYSTEM AND IMMUNE PROTECTION SYSTEM 219 648 317 918

*Fig. 1 Organs of the immune system 214 317 498 817:*

1 – adenoids 471 219 319 819
2 – palatine tonsils 428 641 478 591
3 – thoracic lymphatic duct 514 715 914 815
4 – subclavian vein 598 317 898 214
5 – lymph nodes 514 317 219 419
6 – spleen 548 711 918 321
7 – Peyer's patches 598 721 398 641
8 – small intestine 528 317 428 717
9 – red bone marrow 598 492 319 016
10 – lymphatic vessels 598 064 571 389
11 – right lymphatic duct 418 481 499 164
12 – thymus (thymus) 481 914 319 814
13 – Colon 591 488 898 217
14 – appendix 529 317 899 228

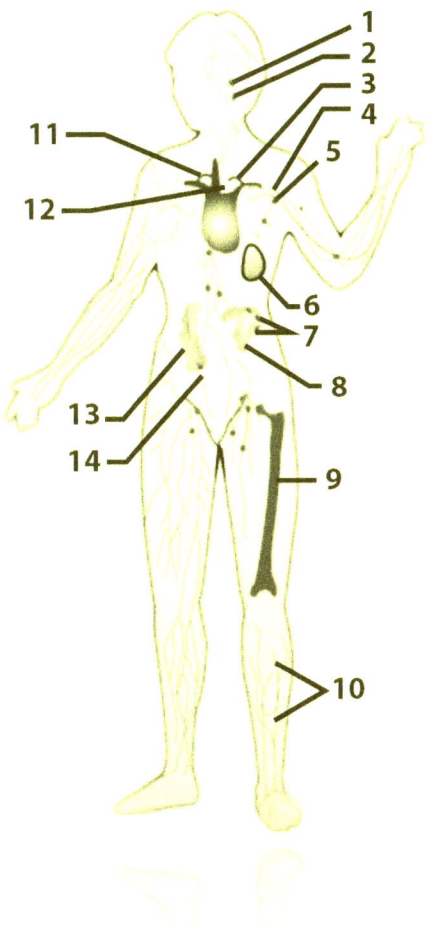

## Central organs of blood formation and immune defense 416 489 319 641

*Fig. 2 Red marrow 497 214 218 641:*

1 – stem cell 451 618 719 481
2 – platelets 649 317 498 714
3 – erythrocyte 214 719 319 818
4 – monocyte 519 671 319 648
5 – lymphocyte 516 318 948 714
6 – basophils 319 648 719 814
7 – eosinophil 549 316 718 491
8 – nsytrofil 467 589 891 648
9 – red (blood-forming) marrow 497 214 218 641
10 – feeding artery 641 849 317 914

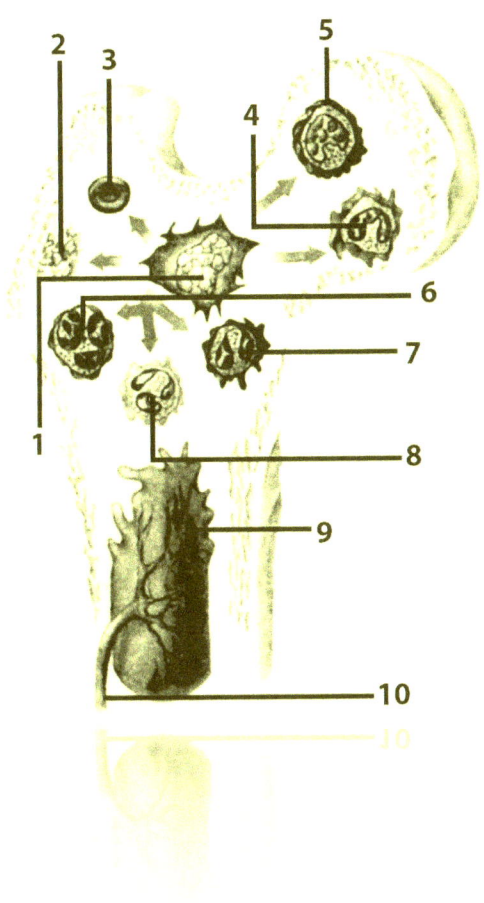

***Fig. 3 lobules of the thymus***
***(thymus gland) (structure) 519 713 219 498:***

I – cortical substance 519 648 219714

II – medullar substance 319 498 516 814

1 – capsule 598 317 948 567

2 – septum 968 319 594 217

3 – macrophage 947 368 249 714

4 – cortical epithelial cell (cell - nurse) 549 361 897 217

5 – cortical layer thymocyte 564 891 218 647

6 – medullary epithelial cell 574 016 217 498

7 – dendritic epithelial cell 598 671 390 149

8 – thymocyte of medulla 531 649 174 061

9 – body of thymus gland 914 864 719 472

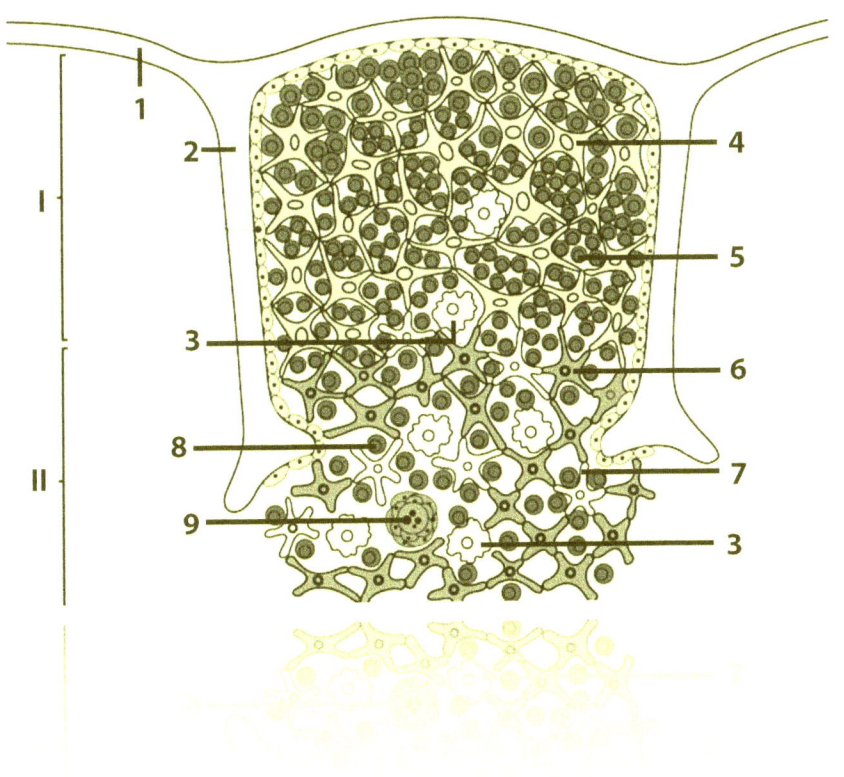

© Грабовой Г.П. 2002

**Peripheral organs of blood formation and immune defense 794 916 219 481**

*Fig. 4 Spleen (structure) 548 711 918 321:*

1 – fibrous tunic 589 491 317 548
2 – spleen trabecula 317 489 896 104
3 – lymphoid follicles of the spleen 517 218 496 471
4 – venous sinuses 594 328 697 541
5 – white pulp 589 674 198 491
6 – red pulp 589 671 318 494

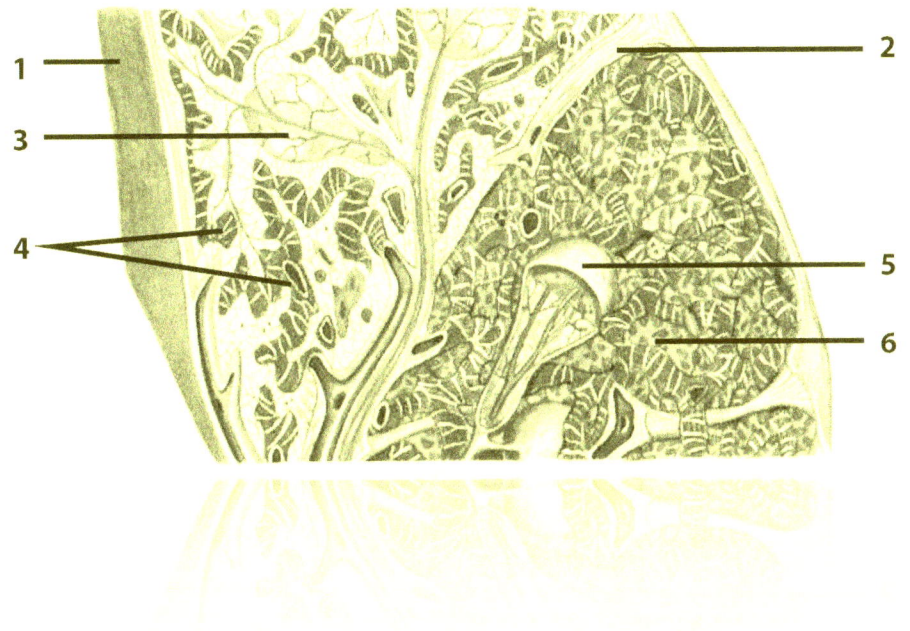

*Fig. 5 Structure of the lymph node 591 148 319 888:*
1 – capsule 519 848 718 949
2 – trabecula 518 716 918 317
3 – cross bar 898 749 219 317
4 – cortical substance 519 421 319 281
5 – follicles 898 715 984 355
6 – afferent lymphatic vessels 598 741 288 511
7 – medullary substance 498 641 319 817
8 – efferent lymphatic vessels 512 789 319 489
9 – the gate of lymph node 598 681 724 918

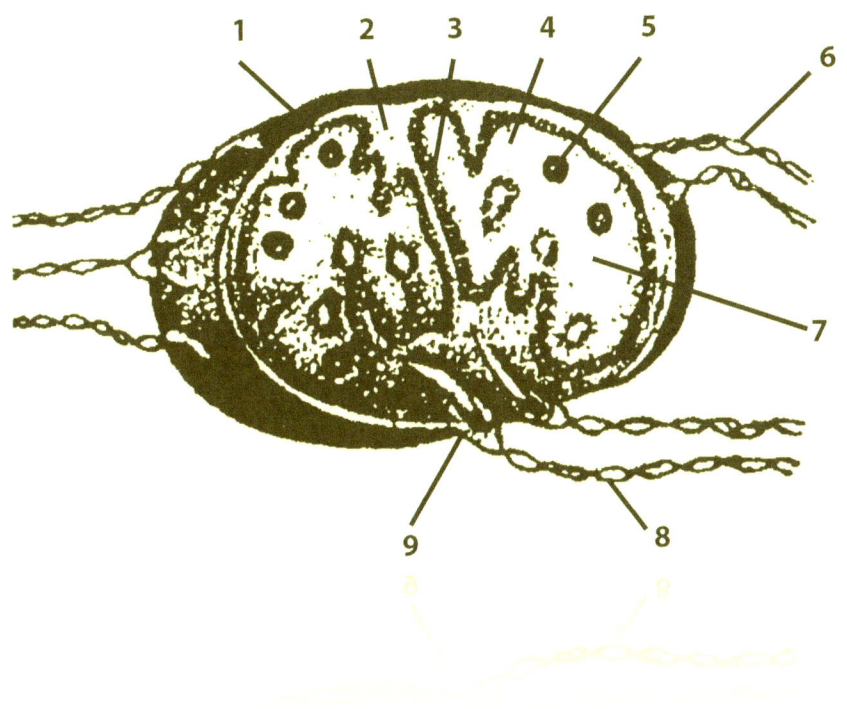

**Single of mucous membranes immune system**
**674 981 219 496**

*Fig. 6 palatine tonsil (located in the oral cavity) 514 218 319 671:*
1 – palatine tonsils 514 218 319 671

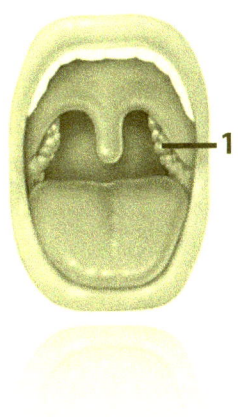

*Fig. 7 palatine tonsil (structure) 514 218 319 671:*

1 – lacunas 894 316 548 917
2 – lymphatic follicles 598 641 317 214
3 – the opening of lacunas 349 548 671 214

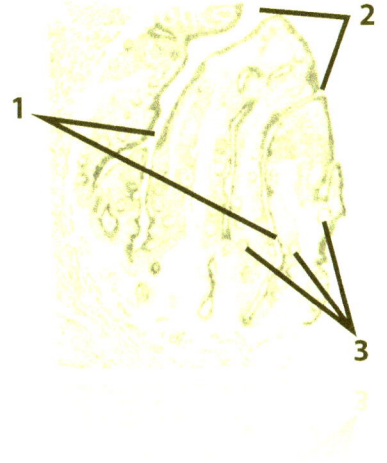

***Fig. 8 lymphoid nodules***
***(in the wall of the appendix) 319 648 317 498:***

1 – wall of the appendix 217 214 218 641
2 – lymphoid nodules 319 648 317 498
3 – epithelium  218 491 016 648

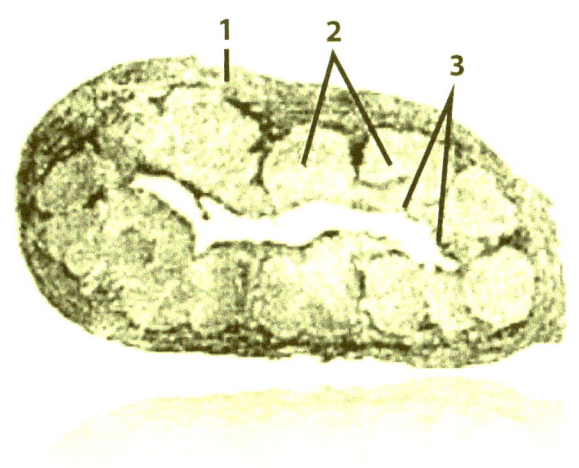

*Fig. 9 Lymphoid nodules and lymphoid plaque in the wall of the small intestine 249 317 498 641:*
1 – lymphoid nodules 548 547 198 678
2 – lymphoid plaque 589 641 948 581

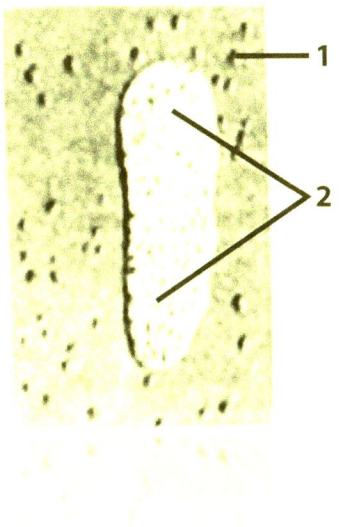

*Fig. 10 antigen-presenting cells (APC) 598 647 319 591:*
I – Langerhans cell 548 491 619 891
1 – Langerhans cell 548 491 619 891
2 – keratinocytes 516 891 719 478
3 – epidermis 598 718 889 888
4 – basement membrane 689 497 597 814
II – follicular dendritic cell 594 716 219 819
III – interdigital cell 548 217 319 471
IV – dendritic cell of multiplication centers 549 621 891 719

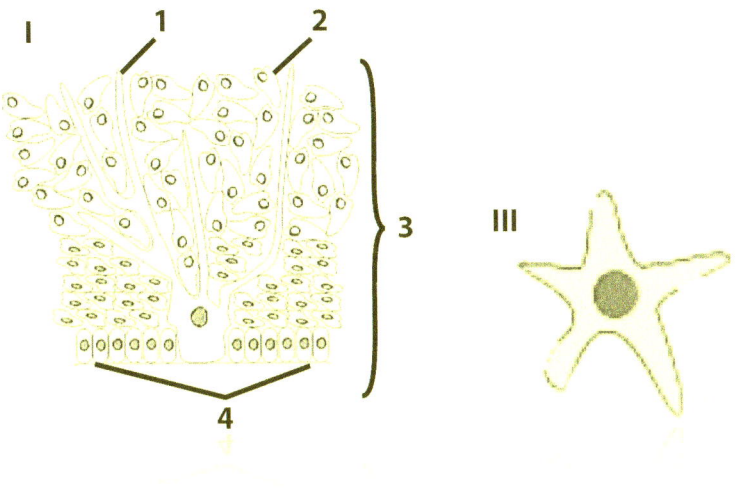

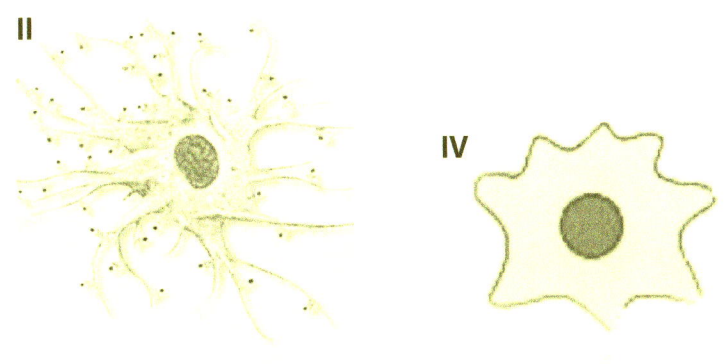

31

© Грабовой Г.П. 2002

**BLOOD CELLS 549681219717**

***Fig. 11 red blood cell 467 198 219 814:***
1 – blood reticulocyte (immature red blood cell) 691 218 498 514
2 – red blood cells 467 198 219 814

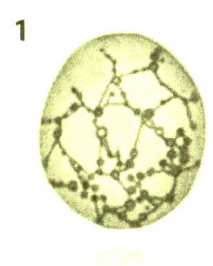

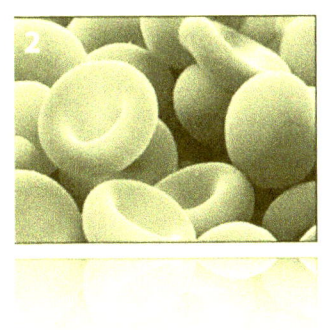

© Грабовой Г.П. 2002

***Fig. 12 erythrogenesis 489 617 519 318:***

1 – erythroblast 589 649 218 717
2 – pronormocyte 218 719 814 798
3 – basophilic normocyte 496 198 217 248
4 – ortohromny normocyte 496 814 219 817
5 – polychromatic normocyte 598 694 197 281
6 – erythrocyte 214 719 319 818

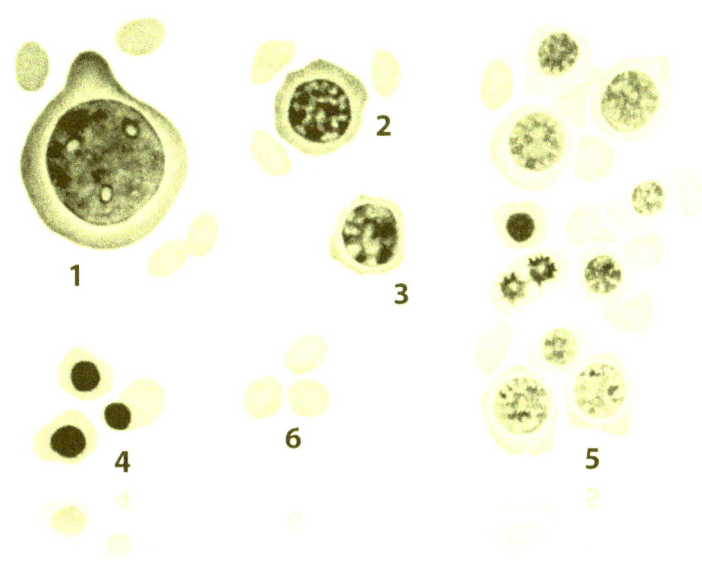

*Fig. 13 thrombocytopoiesis 481 249 016 914:*

1 – megacarioblast 894 316 218 516
2 – Promegakaryocyte 481 216 318 491
3 – megakaryocyte 471 218 694 271
4 – platelets 649 317 498 714

**Thrombopoietin 890 648 019 312**

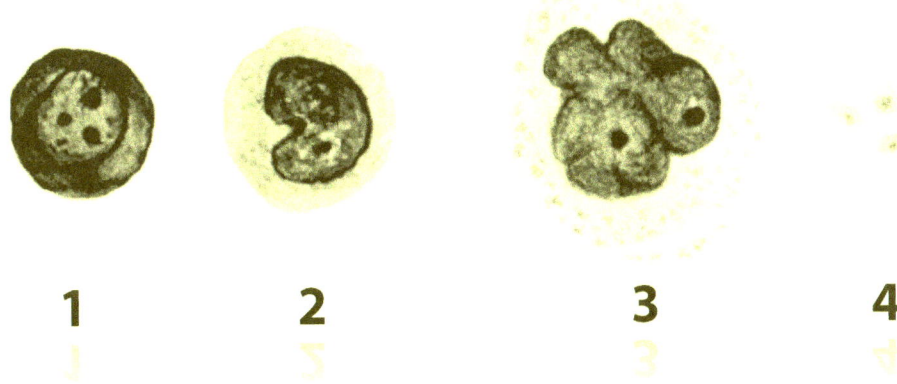

1   2   3   4

© Грабовой Г.П. 2002

**Leukocytes 694 218 574 271**
**Agranulocytes 548 274 298 641**

*Fig. 14 lymphocytopoiesis 648 041 298 471:*

I – B – lymphocytes 518 541 316 218
1 – B – lymphoblast 316 491 519 618
2 – immature B – lymphocyte 518 491 217 496
3 – mature B – lymphocyte 498 164 019 981
II – T – lymphocytes 467 198 964 217
1 – T – lymphoblast 316 514 816 274
2 – immature T – lymphocyte 619 754 218 316
3 – mature T – lymphocyte 689 148 686 217

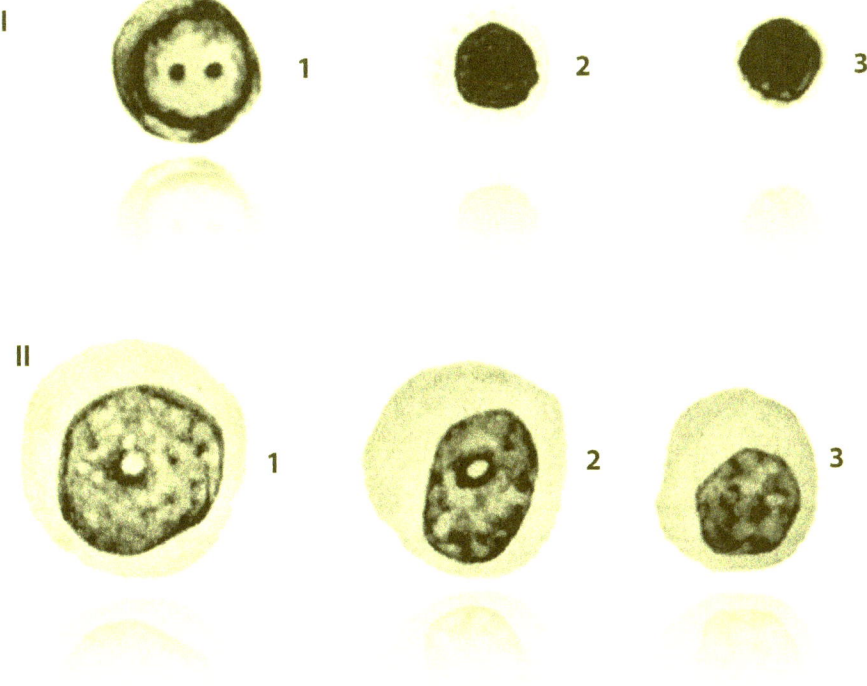

© Грабовой Г.П. 2002

***Fig. 15 monocytopoiesis. Formation of
monocytes and macrophages 496 514 218 471:***
1 – monocytoblast 319 471 819 498
2 – promonocyte 619 814 516 714
3 – monocyte 519 671 319 648
4 – macrophage 947 368 249 714

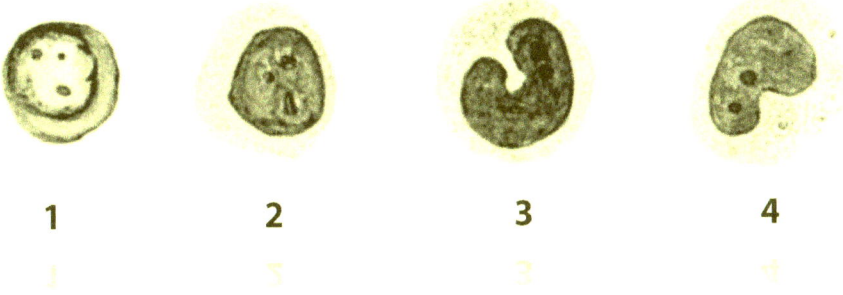

1 2 3 4

# Granulocytes 918 547 219 714

*Fig. 16 granulocytopoiesis 214 617 218 549:*

I – formation of basophilic granulocytes 584 316 318 491
1 – myeloblast 549 641 894 317
2 – progranulocyte 496 548 219 641
3 – medullocell 517 219 498 641
4 – metamyelocyte 894 216 219 891
5 – band-form basophils 217 214 619 061
6 – segment-nuclear basophils 648 918 818 491
II – the formation of eosinophilic granulocytes 496 549 718 546
1 – myeloblast 549 641 894 317
2 – progranulocyte 496 548 219 641
3 – medullocell 517 219 498 641
4 – metamyelocyte 894 216 219 891
5 – band-form eosinophil 549 648 598 748
6 – segmentonuclear eosinophil 548 461 719 496
III – formation of neutrophilic granulocytes 564 581 498 641
1 – myeloblast 549 641 894 317
2 – progranulocyte 496 548 219 641
3 – medullocell 517 219 498 641
4 – metamyelocyte 894 216 219 891
5 – band-form neutrophil 568 191 219 714
6 – segmentonuclear neutrophil 894 961 068 971

I

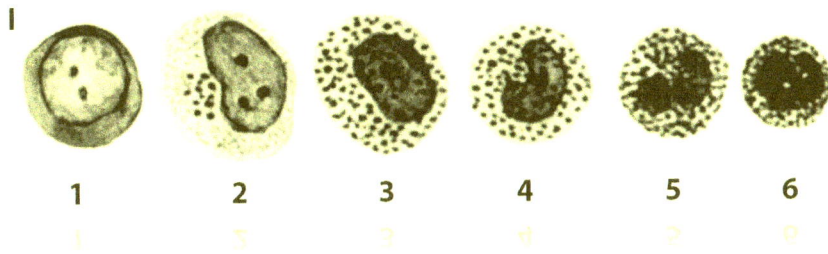

1  2  3  4  5  6

II

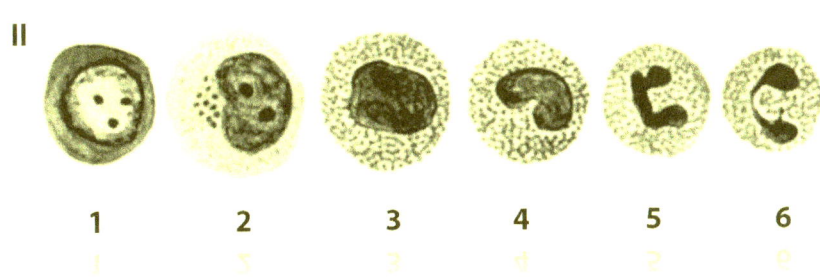

1  2  3  4  5  6

III

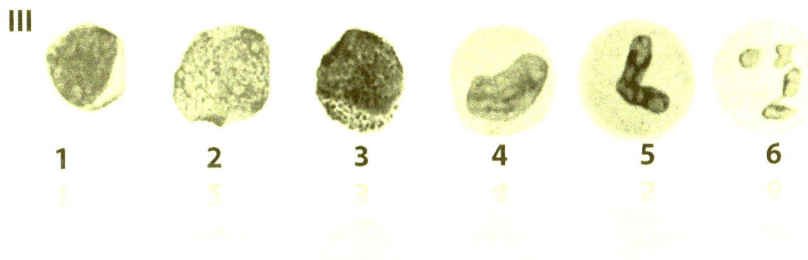

1  2  3  4  5  6

## DENTOALVEOLAR SYSTEM
## 216 548 219 716

### Facial bones of the skull 219 715 819 815

***Fig. 17 The upper jaw***
*(view from the lateral side) 519 371 919 811:*

1 – orbital surface 398 216 718 226

2 – infraorbital groove 319 717 819 227

3 – zygomatic process 419 312 214 222

4 – alveolar openings 214 712 814 229

5 – infratemporal surface 538 722 918 222

6 – anterior surface 548 888 019 648

7 – fang pit 539 717 819 317

8 – acanthion 529 513 919 813

9 – body of the maxilla 548712 818 212

10 – nasal notch 548 716 298 444

11 – infraorbital canal 319 717 819 217

12 – infraorbital foramen 489 061 298 541

13 – zygomaticomaxillary seam 214 711 898 211

14 – frontal process 590 421 019 481

15 – lacrimal edge 548 884 918 888

16 – infraorbital edge 512 219 312 919

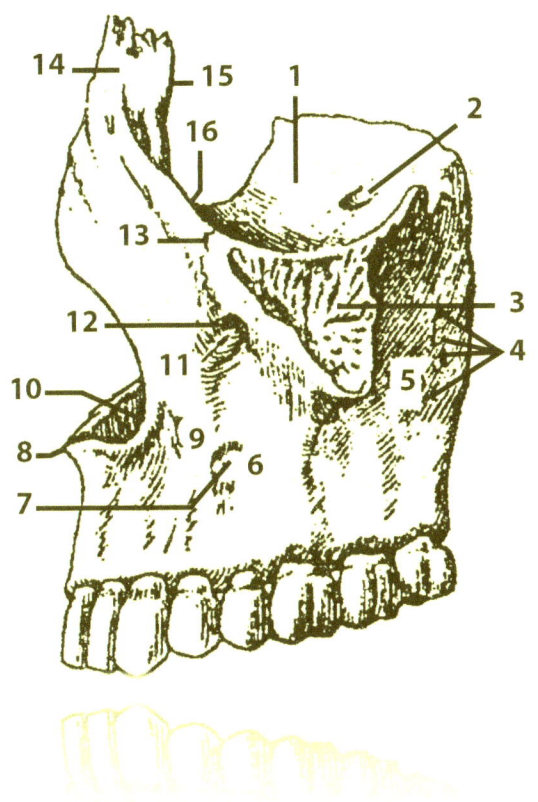

***Fig. 18 The upper jaw (left)***
***(view from the medial side) 421 718 911 328:***

1 – frontal process 590 421 019 481
2 – nasal surface 598 648 319 711
3 – acanthion 529 513 919 813
4 – pterygoid-palatine groove 428 321 814 221
5 – maxillary (Highmore) sinus 519 321 814 471

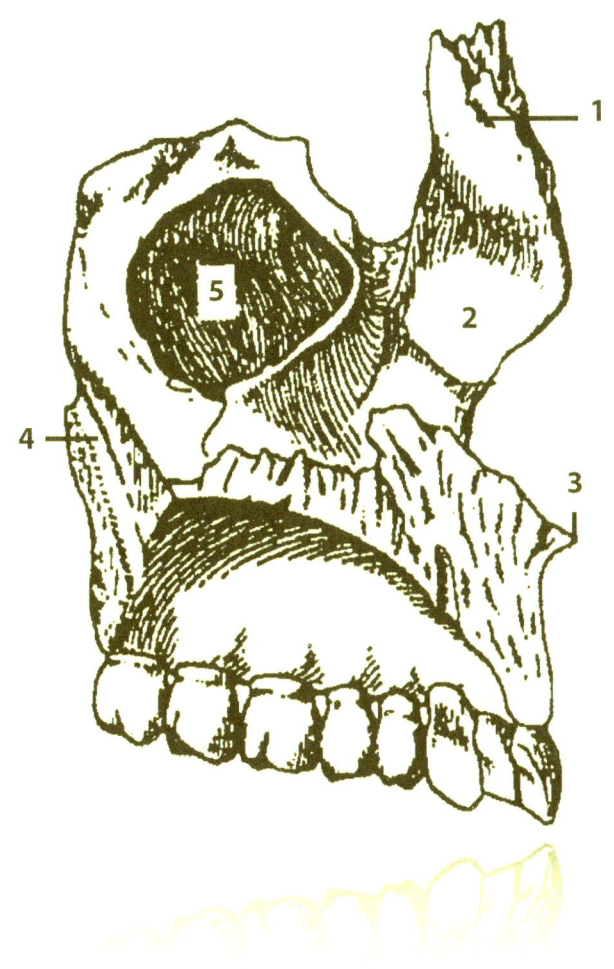

© Грабовой Г.П. 2002

***Fig. 19 Lower jaw 514 712 814 312:***

1 – head of mandible 548 321 848 721
2 – pterygoid fossa 519 317 919 007
3 – neck of mandible 319 814 919 714
4, 5 – the branches of mandible 518 317 918 001
6 – the angle of mandible 548 219 289 008
7 – channel of mandible 009 217 319 227
8 – temporal ridge 418 317 228 227
9 – opening of mandible 489 201 319 871
10 – coronoid process 528 317 918 228
11 – incisure of mandible 419 317 819 828
12 – condylar process 891 319 898 789

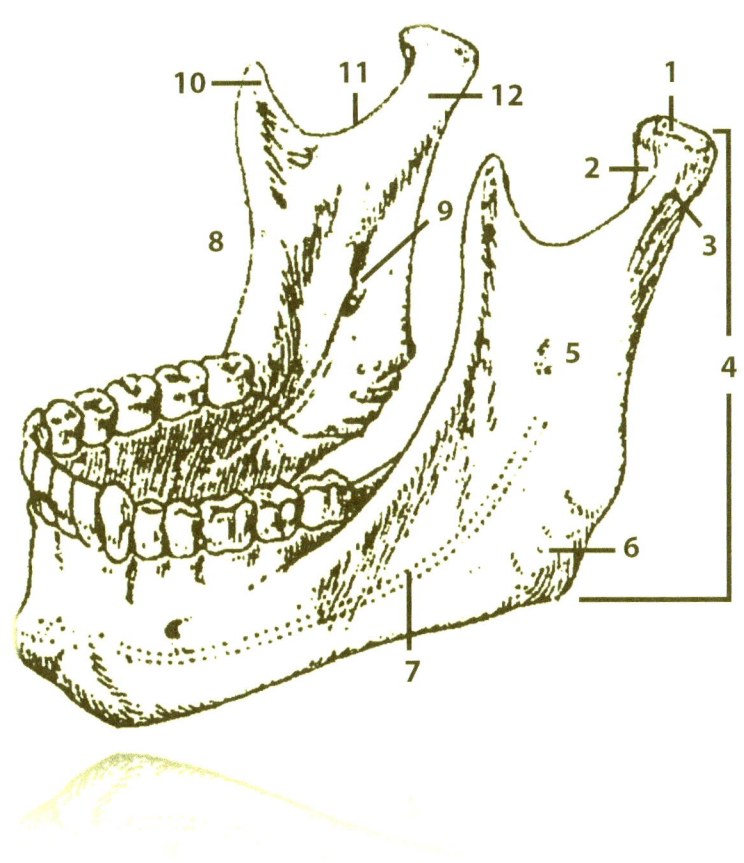

*Fig. 20 Osteo-cartilaginous skeleton of external nose 948 547 219 641:*

1 – nasal bone 518 314 818 214
2 – minor cartilage of the nose wings 916 814 219 618
3 – greater cartilage of wing of the nose 719 316 219 494
4 – accessory nasal cartilage 989 617 318 641
5 – lateral cartilage 289 671 318 491

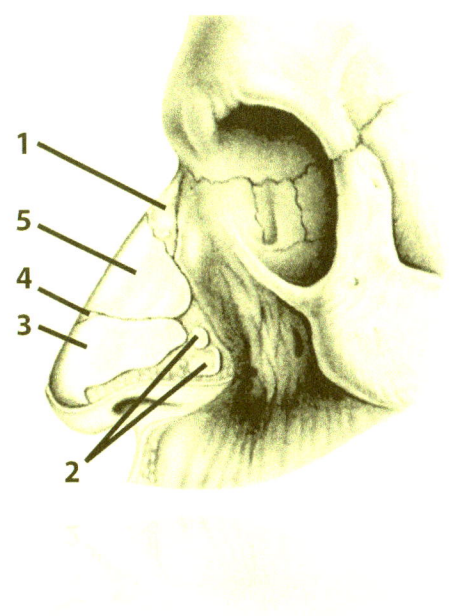

*Fig. 21 The nasal bone 518 314 818 214:*
1 – internasal suture 514 314 218 578
2 – opening of nasal bone 316 581 314 891
3 – free edge 598 641 719 471

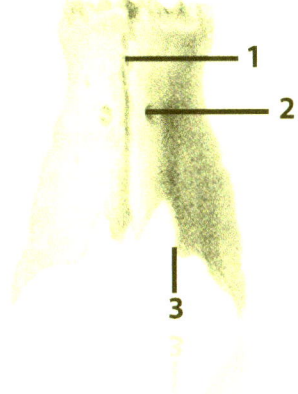

*Fig. 22 Inferior turbinate 478 218 918 217:*

A – Exterior view

B – interior view

1 – lacrimal process 548 671 219 491

2 – slatted process 491 897 319 648

3 – maxillary process 589 671 918 491

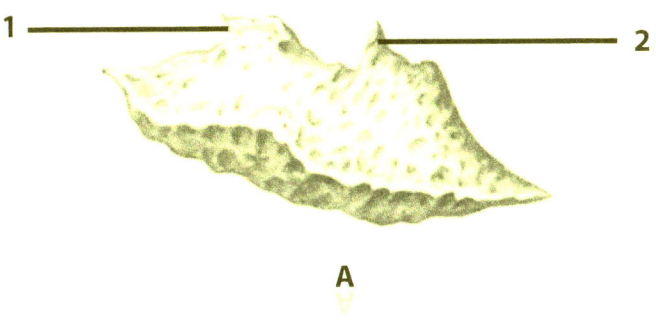

**А**

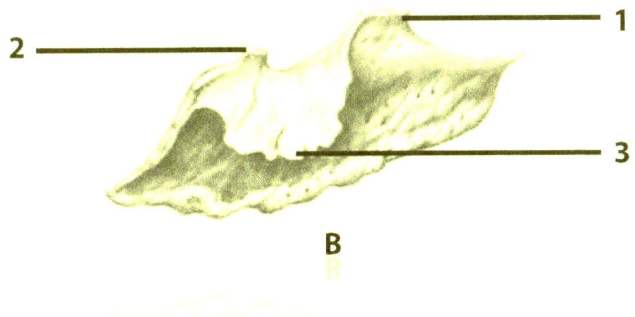

**В**

***Fig. 23 Zygomatic bone 899 817 818 317:***
1 – frontal process 590 421 019 481
2 – orbital surface 398 216 718 226
3 – zygomaticoorbital foramen 481 467 219 891
4 – lateral surface 948 541 698 718
5 – temporal process 694 171 219 548

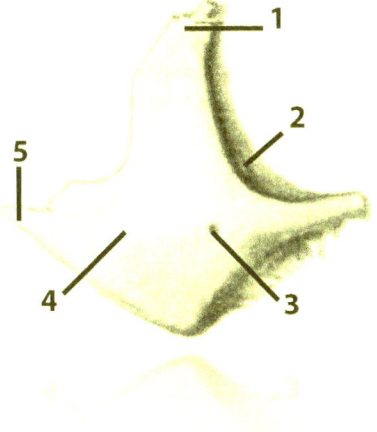

*Fig. 24 Palatine bone (right) (exterior view) 641 214 918 516:*
1 – wedge-shaped appendage 584 218 649 317
2 – wedge-palatal incisure 549 641 219 811
3 – orbital process 549 674 317 581
4 – perpendicular plate 648 171 219 549
5 – horizontal plate 691 814 217 318
6 – greater palatine groove 394 698 598 714
7 – pyramidal process 691 218 514 317

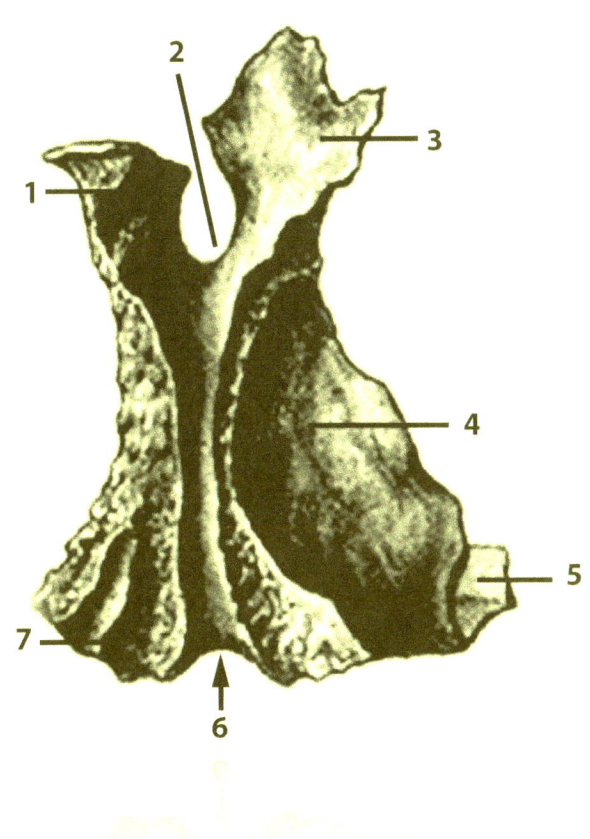

*Fig. 25 palatine bone, right (inside view) 649 314 219 516:*
1 – orbital process 549 674 317 581
2 – wedge-palatal notch 549 612 814 914
3 – wedge-shaped appendage 584 218 649 317
4 – pyramidal process 691 218 514 317
5 – horizontal plate 691 814 217 318
6 – perpendicular plate 648 171 219 549
7 – conchal crest 698 314 218 597
8 – ethmoidal crest 467 214 909 814

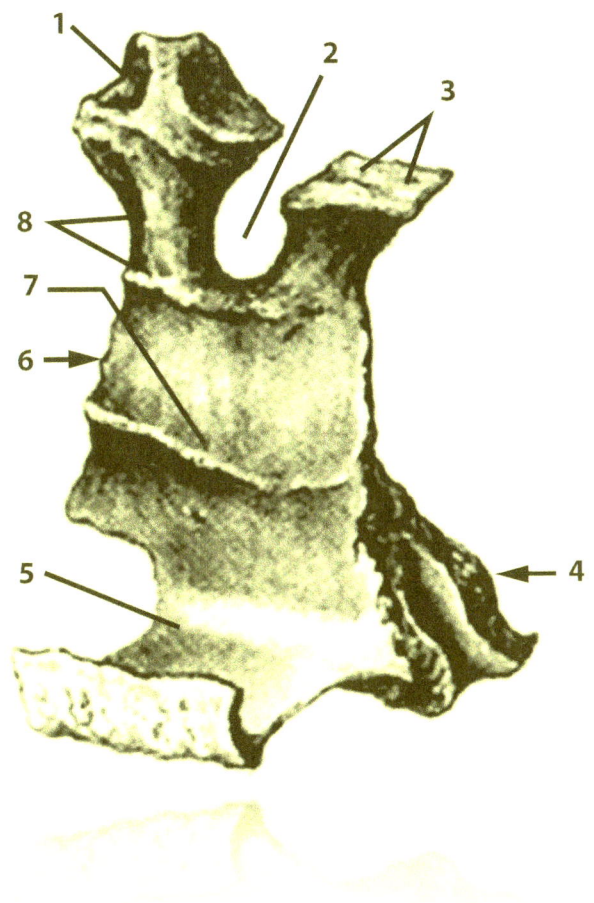

## Teeth 698 314 819 516

*Fig. 26 General structure of the tooth:*

1 – crown of the tooth 319 594 938 716
2 – neck of the tooth 364 891 219 491
3 – the root of the tooth 368 549 188 794
4 – dental papilla 364 198 501 248
5 – dental groove 601 549 906 714
6 – root apex 594 315 498 515
7 – tooth enamel 618 374 898 161
8 – dentin, tooth substance 548 314 819 716
9 – dental pulp, the pulp of the tooth 316 481 219 649
10 – crown pulp 318 691 378 549
11 – pulp of root 471 649 398 591
12 – canal of tooth root 894 160 498 497
13 – Cement 314 861 219 492

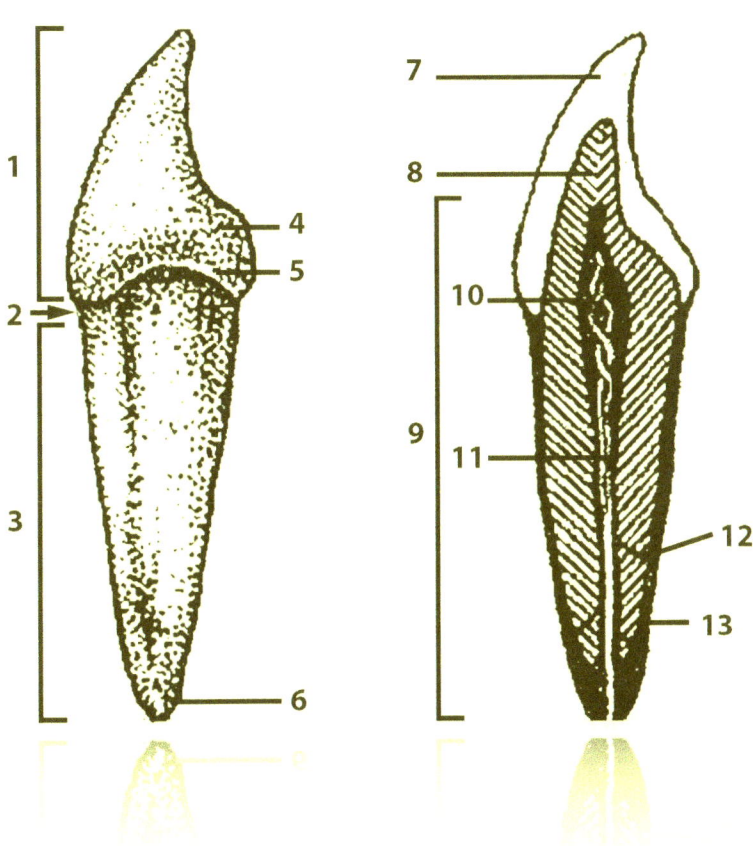

***Fig. 27 The structure of the tooth and surrounding tissues:***
a – crown of tooth 319 594 938 716
b – root 368 549 188 794
1 –  fissure 546 218 319 491
2 – tooth enamel 618 374 898 161
3 – dentin 548 314 819 716
4 – pulp 316 481 219 649
5 – gingival groove 518 316 549 471
6 – gum 479 168 318 517
7 – periodontium 482 316 219 491
8 – nerve fibers 478 514 219 671
9 – arterial vessels 894 378 214 316
10 – venous vessels 319 681 214 784
11 – Cement of root 698 541 349 172
12 – canal of tooth root 894 160 498 497
13 – apical foramen 485 694 319 718
14 – jaw bone 318 549 468 019
15 – main neurovascular bundle 589 314 694 817

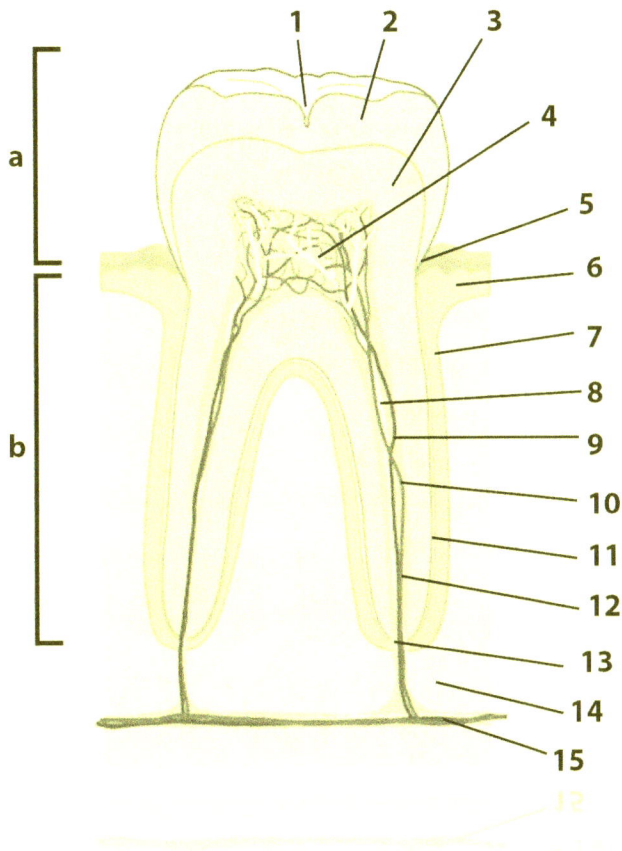

***Fig. 28 Structure of maxillodental segments:***

1 – the tooth-gum fibers 461 519 819 479
2 – alveolar walls 584 216 319 481
3 – dento-alveolar fibers 584 167 219 491
4 – alveolar-gingival branch 479 581 316 594
5 – periodontal vessels 891 478 219 641
6 – artery and veins of jaw 984 517 219 648
7 – tooth branch of nerve 794 281 298 641
8 – the bottom of the alveoli 514 368 791 498
9 – tooth root 368 549 188 794
10 – neck of the tooth 364 891 219 491
11 – crown of the tooth 319 594 938 716
12 – interdental (interroot) fibers 314 548 914 281

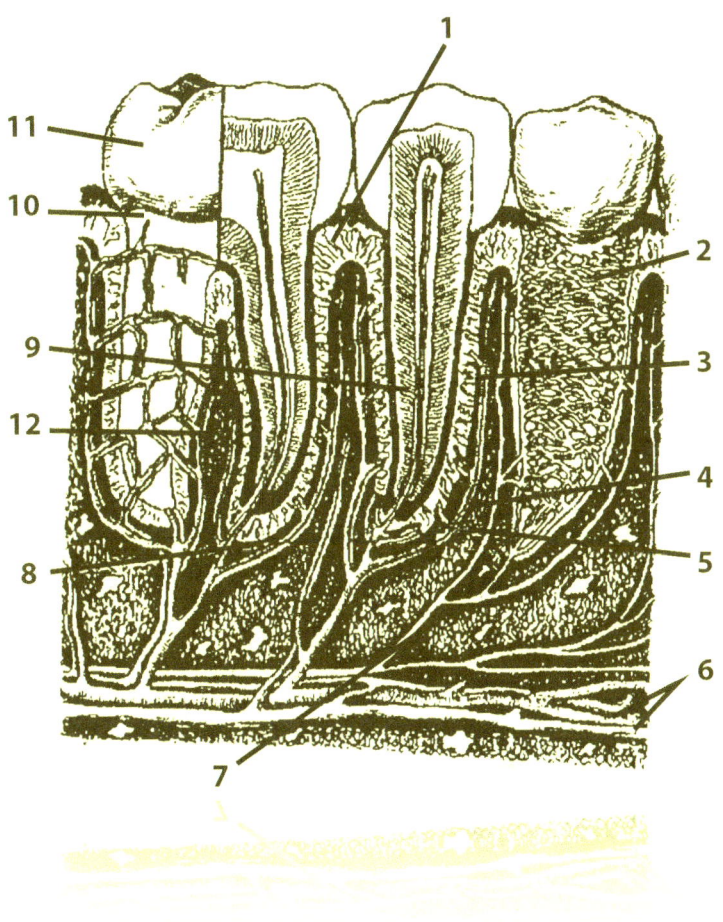

*Fig. 29 teeth of the upper and mandibulas, permanent (right) 594 819 498 716:*

1 – upper molars (left to right) 648 517 216 318
    - Upper azzle tooth, tricuspid (molar) III 498 516 318 914
    - Upper azzle teeth (molar)  II 548 491 478 694
    - Upper azzle teeth (molar) I 369 481 319 478
2 – alveolar elevations of the upper jaw 594 318 498 614
3 – minor upper molars (left to right) 694 317 219 498
    - Upper bicuspid tooth (bicuspid) II 378 498 514 916
    - Upper bicuspid tooth (bicuspid)  I 614 218 598 781
4 – alveolar process of the upper jaw 986 149 318 518
5 – upper canine 471 891 016 498
6 – upper incisors (left to right) 519 671 918 549
    - Lateral incisor 549 691 718 548
    - Medial incisor 914 501 604 981
7 – alveolar part of the mandible 519 317 218 498
8 – lower medial incisor 584 716 914 219
9 – lower lateral incisor 989 718 514 601
10 – lower canine 589 318 499 164
11 – lower bicuspid tooth (bicuspid) I 518 016 949 148
12 – lower bicuspid tooth (bicuspid) II 514 817 316 498
13 – lower molar tooth (molar) I 518 495 319 816
14 – lower molar teeth (molar) II 519 814 317 984
15 – lower molar teeth (molar) III 541 219 016 898
16 – mandibula 514 712 814 312

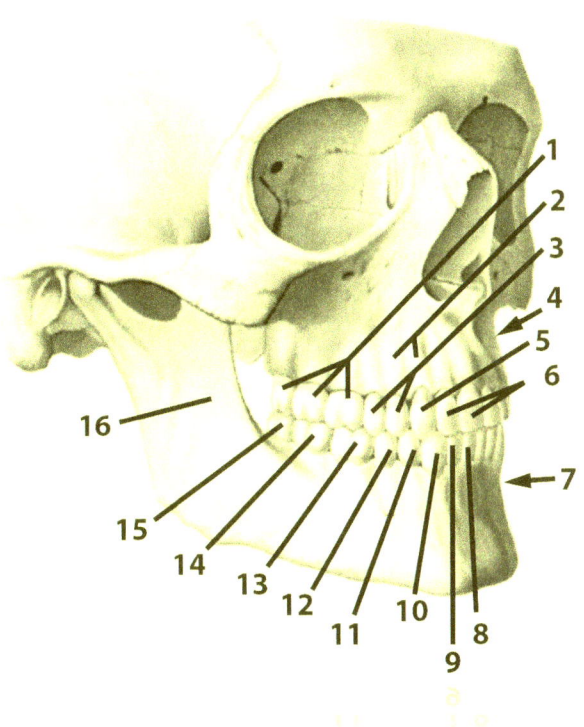

***Fig. 30 The medial upper incisor (right) 914 501 604 981:***
1 – vestibular surface 514 568 219 317
2 – mesial surface 314 894 319 892
3 – lingual surface 598 471 219 648
4 – interior view of a tooth in the vestibulo-lingual plane 914 818 016 594
5 – interior view of the tooth in the medio-distal plane 317 648 519 819
6 – cutting surface 498 317 219 491
7 – canal of tooth root 584 641 718 547
8 – pulp of root 910 849 189 647
9 – pulp of crown 319 648 519 987

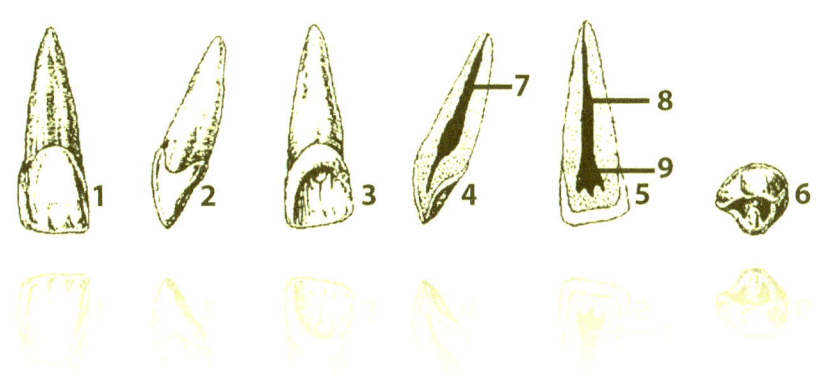

*Fig. 31 The lateral upper incisor (right) 549 691 718 548:*
1 – vestibular surface 514 916 917 518
2 – mesial surface 498 614 819 594
3 – lingual surface 718 594 319 681
4 – interior view of a tooth in the vestibulo-lingual plane 594 716 918 916
5 – interior view of the tooth in the medio-distal plane 549 817 394 617
6 – cutting surface 581 349 619 817
7 – canal of tooth root 398 641 594 818
8 – pulp of root 318 691 219 348
9 – pulp of crown 819 601 698 149

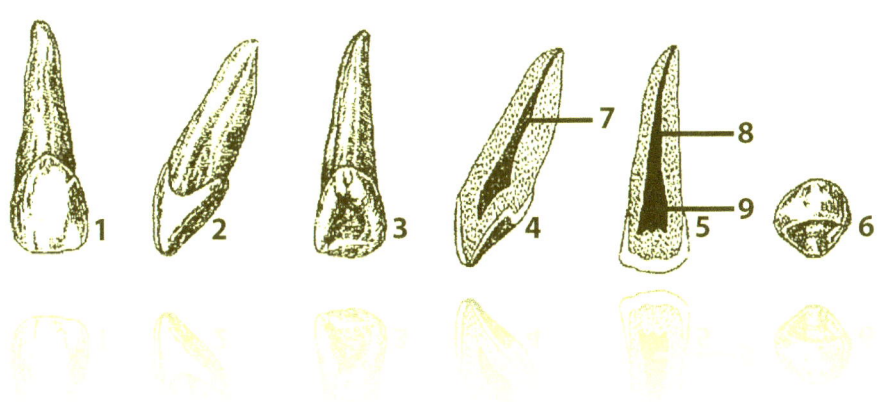

***Fig. 32 The medial lower incisor (right) 584 716 914 219:***
1 – vestibular surface 496 198 216 291
2 – mesial surface 481 478 594 316
3 – lingual surface 894 594 168 917
4 – interior view of a tooth in the vestibulo-lingual plane 198 649 319 641
5 – interior view of the tooth in the medio-distal plane 894 167 318 491
6 – cutting surface 364 517 219 581
7 – canal of tooth root 318 694 369 471
8 – pulp of root 949 516 817 919
9 – pulp of crown 949 190 649 871

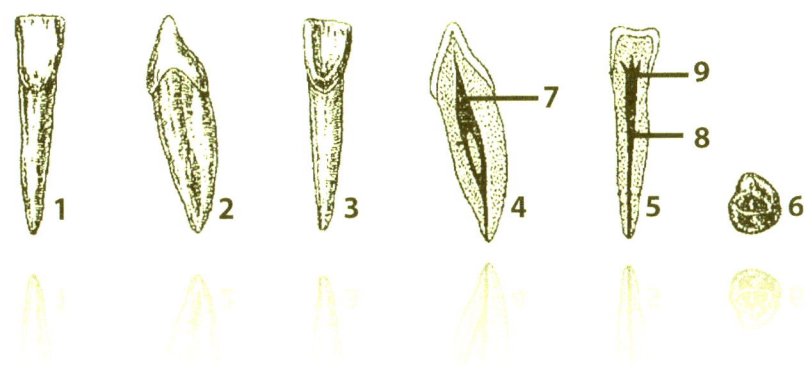

***Fig. 33 lower lateral incisor (right) 989 718 514 601:***

1 – vestibular surface 694 187 219 471
2 – mesial surface 468 271 398 497
3 – lingual surface 894 561 219 718
4 – interior view of a tooth in the vestibulo-lingual plane 584 617 219 714
5 – interior view of the tooth in the medio-distal plane 689 318 514 712
6 – cutting surface 799 814 218 564
7 – canal of tooth root 368 194 371 894
8 – pulp of root 964 718 519 498
9 – pulp of crown 698 318 564 917

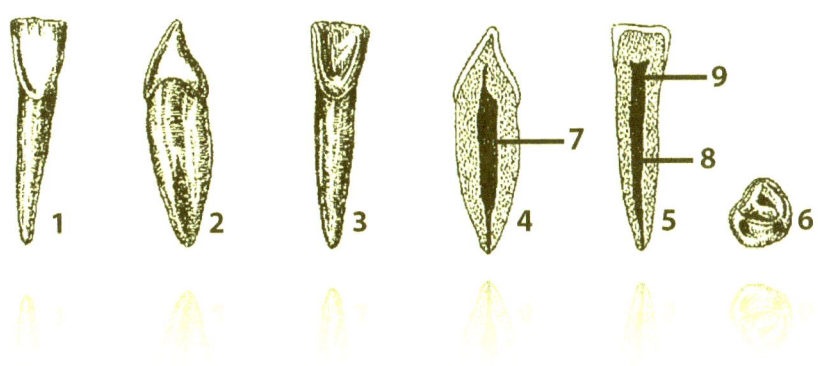

*Fig. 34 upper canine (right) 471 891 016 498:*

1 – vestibular surface 468 716 519 498
2 – mesial surface 618 471 219 472
3 – lingual surface 549 316 218 581
4 – interior view of a tooth in the vestibulo-lingual plane 918 516 319 491
5 – interior view of the tooth in the medio-distal plane 819 604 916 989
6 – cutting surface 641 519 318 491
7 – canal of tooth root 384 591 689 374
8 – pulp of root 989 618 054 132
9 – pulp of crown 968 108 604 271

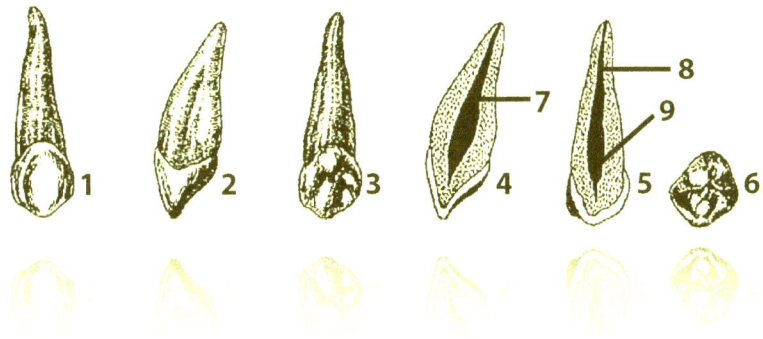

***Fig. 35 The lower canine (right) 589 318 499 164:***
1 – vestibular surface 698 318 514 217
2 – mesial surface 319 481 318 641
3 – lingual surface 948 564 008 904
4 – interior view of a tooth in the vestibulo-lingual plane 368 014 218 548
5 – interior view of the tooth in the medio-distal plane 648 781 949 064
6 – cutting surface 546 981 941 568
7 – canal of tooth root 714 801 498 541
8 – pulp of root 398 614 718 581
9 – pulp of crown 689 841 598 671

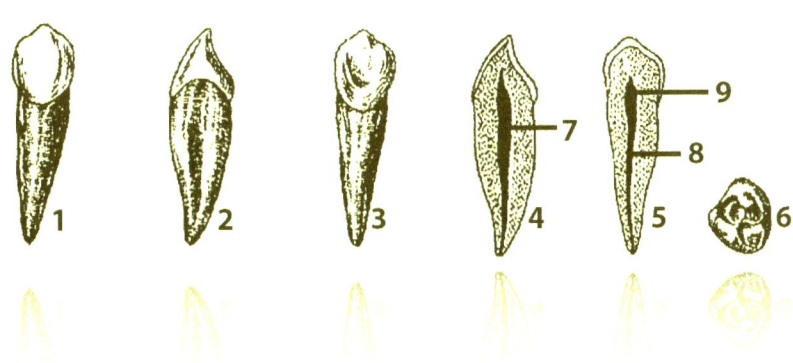

*Fig. 36 The first upper premolar (right) 614 218 598 781:*
1 – vestibular surface 691 378 594 971
2 – mesial surface 498 617 898 541
3 – lingual surface 894 671 219 818
4 – interior view of a tooth in the vestibulo-lingual plane 594 317 589 171
5 – interior view of the tooth in the medio-distal plane 478 641 219 891
6 – chewing surface 364 810 068 901
7 – canal of tooth root 301 514 609 891
8 – pulp of root 478 514 618 717
9 – pulp of crown 984 018 198 601

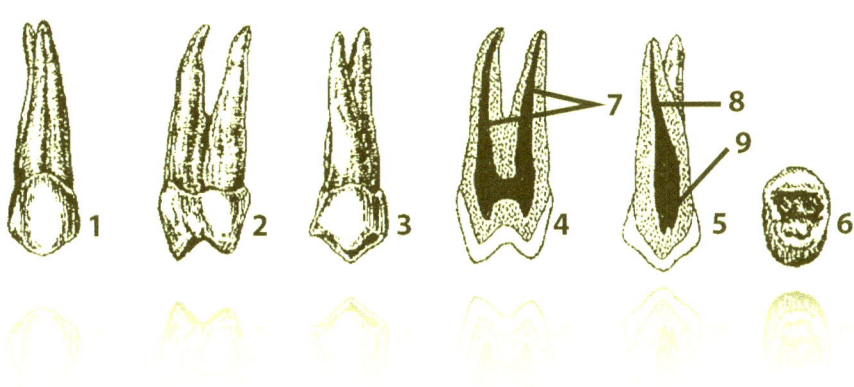

***Fig. 37 Second upper premolar (right) 378 498 514 916:***

1 – vestibular surface 948 561 319 818
2 – mesial surface 319 801 498 561
3 – lingual surface 467 219 498 541
4 – interior view of a tooth in the vestibulo-lingual plane 398 548 589 617
5 – interior view of the tooth in the medio-distal plane 549 819 319 616
6 – chewing surface 389 541 379 818
7 – canal of tooth root 648 546 319 818
8 – pulp of root 894 361 219 012
9 – pulp of crown 064 541 218 317

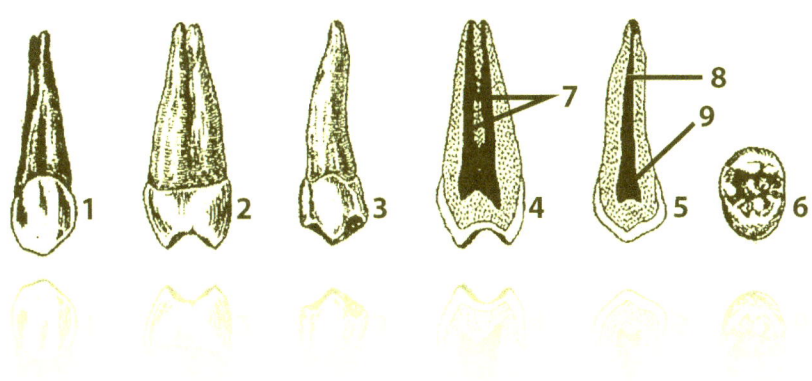

*Fig. 38 The first lower premolar (right) 518 016 949 148:*
1 – vestibular surface 491 679 318 541
2 – mesial surface 549 361 819 497
3 – lingual surface 469 817 318 541
4 – interior view of a tooth in the vestibulo-lingual plane 918 541 219 678
5 – interior view of the tooth in the medio-distal plane 814 319 898 514
6 – chewing surface 518 618 319 714
7 – canal of tooth root 589 491 319 614
8 – pulp of root 214 819 318 617
9 – pulp of crown 914 218 519 641

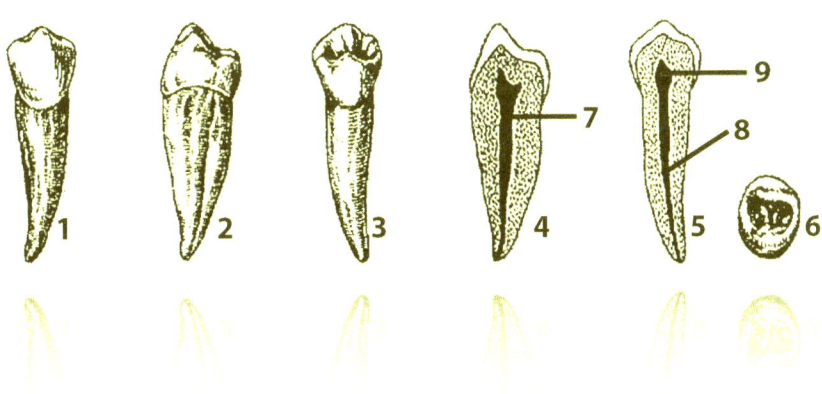

***Fig. 39 Second lower premolar (right) 514 817 316 498:***
1 – vestibular surface 698 517 319 641
2 – mesial surface 498 549 617 218
3 – lingual surface 894 317 218 491
4 – interior view of a tooth in the vestibulo-lingual plane 469 518 519 641
5 – interior view of the tooth in the medio-distal plane 898 416 019 848
6 – chewing surface 841 319 718 491
7 – canal of tooth root 198 741 894 848
8 – pulp of root 168 571 219 491
9 – pulp of crown 371 549 619 814

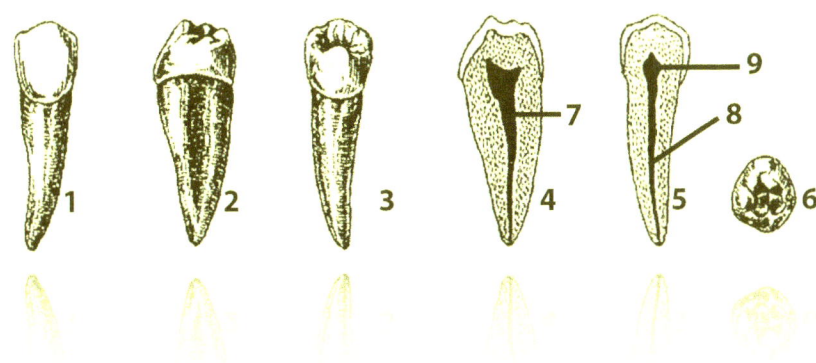

***Fig. 40 First upper molar (right) 369 481 319 478:***
1 – vestibular surface 491 614 718 541
2 – mesial surface 849 516 219 491
3 – lingual surface 684 517 919 486
4 – interior view of a tooth in the vestibulo-lingual plane 584 619 319 814
5 – chewing surface 714 318 519 491
6 – roots of tooth canals 584 168 319 817
7 – pulp of root 849 516 914 971
8 – pulp of crown 318 619 819 498

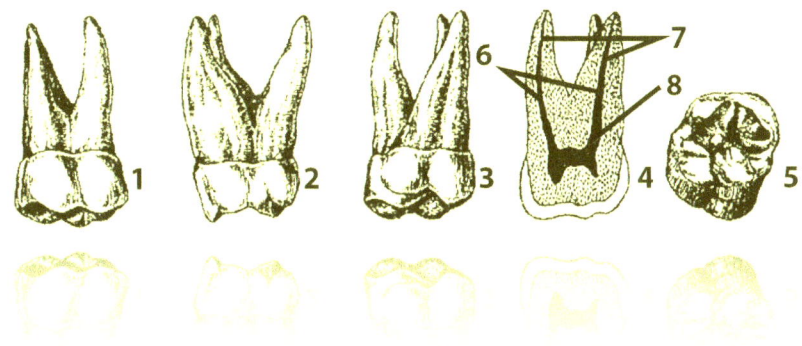

***Fig. 41 Second upper molar (right) 548 491 478 694:***
1 – vestibular surface 984 316 219 491
2 – mesial surface 894 518 319 491
3 – lingual surface 914 816 317 498
4 – interior view of a tooth in the vestibulo-lingual plane 467 548 919 814
5 – chewing surface 214 391 898 491
6 – canal of tooth root 316 598 368 498
7 – pulp of root 648 718 598 647
8 – pulp of crown 894 517 219 498

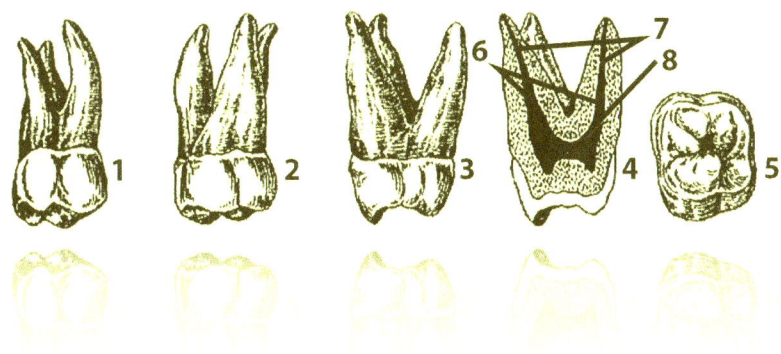

*Fig. 42 Third upper molar (right) 498 516 318 914:*
1 – vestibular surface 618 317 319 641
2 – mesial surface 689 064 194 818
3 – lingual surface 549 618 598 641
4 – interior view of a tooth in the vestibulo-lingual plane 594 198 574 891
5 – chewing surface 648 591 318 498
6 – canals of tooth roots 491 684 898 718
7 – pulp of root 964 717 988 149
8 – pulp of crown 691 948 584 161

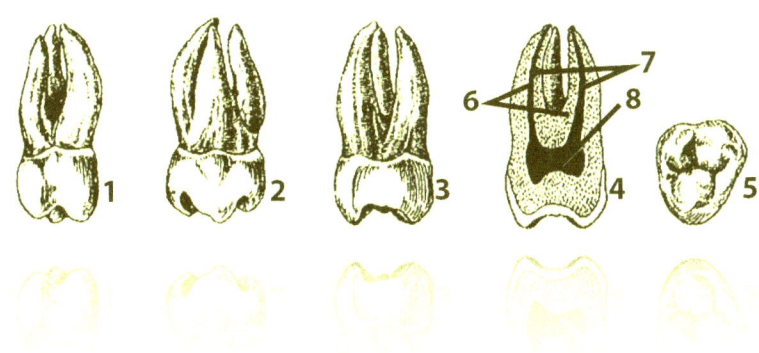

***Fig. 43 First lower molar (right) 518 495 319 816:***
1 – vestibular surface 319 681 519 894
2 – mesial surface 594 895 619 548
3 – lingual surface 694 171 218 541
4 – interior view of a tooth in the vestibulo-lingual plane 549 614 318 541
5 – chewing surface 364 918 598 714
6 – canals of tooth roots 398 617 218 541
7 – pulp of root 368 914 898 516
8 – pulp of crown 319 891 498 516

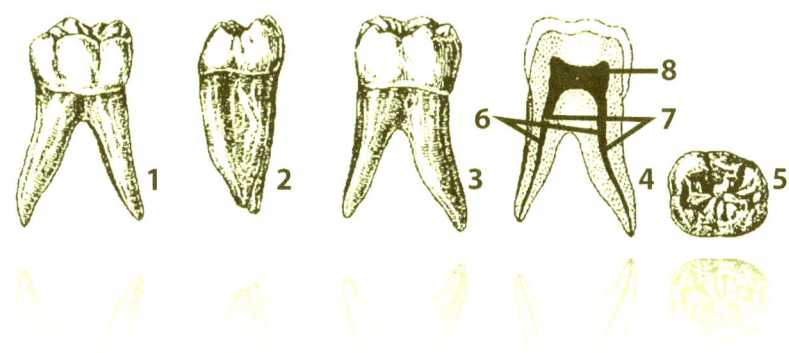

*Fig. 44 Second lower molar (right) 519 814 317 984:*
1 – vestibular surface 419 815 319 641
2 – mesial surface 498 316 318 541
3 – lingual surface 398 814 516 817
4 – interior view of a tooth in the vestibulo-lingual plane 648 512 319 649
5 – chewing surface 504 194 981 369
6 – canals of tooth roots 894 016 598 641
7 – pulp of root 897 491 219 896
8 – pulp of crown 649 197 598 621

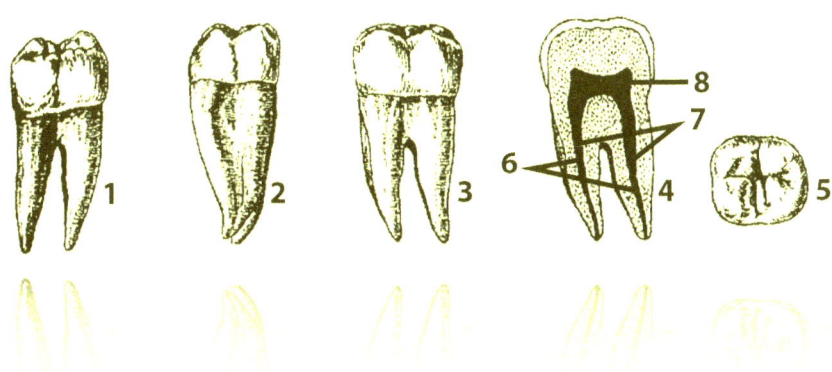

*Fig. 45 Third lower molar (right) 541 219 016 898:*
1 – vestibular surface 617 218 219 491
2 – mesial surface 694 817 219 497
3 – lingual surface 694 181 364 971
4 – interior view of a tooth in the vestibulo-lingual plane 598 564 319 916
5 – chewing surface 948 516 218 949
6 – canals of tooth roots 319 491 819 647
7 – pulp of root 384 161 219 491
8 – pulp of crown 489 516 219 496

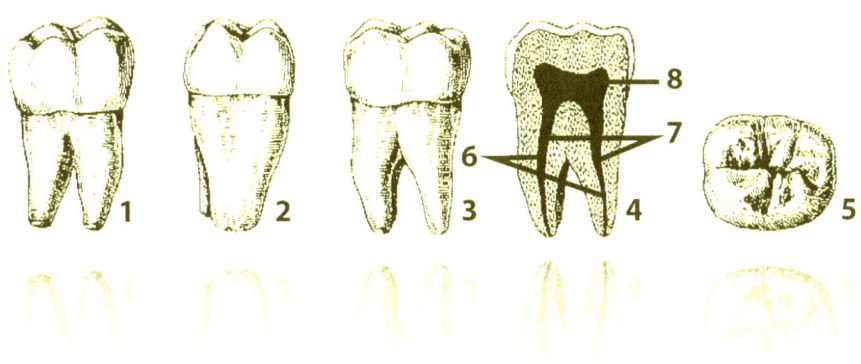

***Fig. 46 Milk incisor, medial, upper (right) 491 518 614 917:***
1 – vestibular surface 549 618 219 814
2 – mesial surface 497 148 684 598
3 – lingual surface 248 379 064 898
4 – cutting surface 491 897 319 648

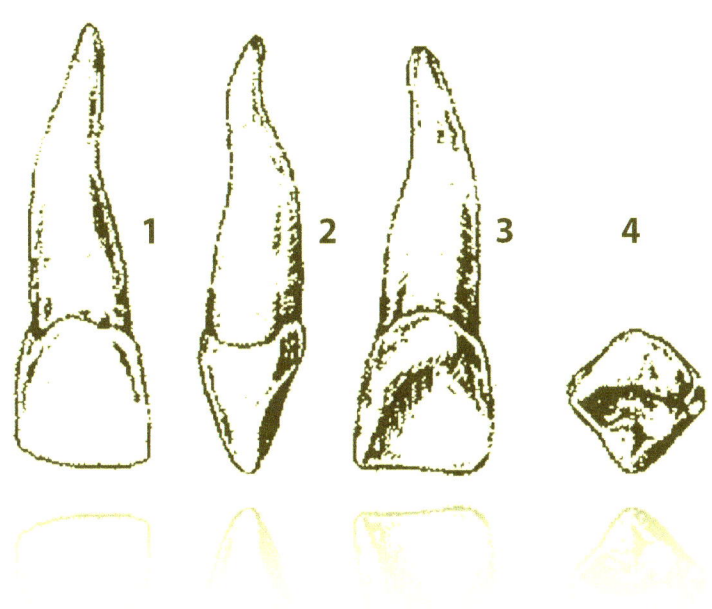

*Fig. 47 Milk incisor, lateral, upper (right) 514 218 919 648:*
1 – vestibular surface 894 161 917 219
2 – mesial surface 619 517 319 498
3 – lingual surface 689 142 398 191
4 – cutting surface 218 589 649 171

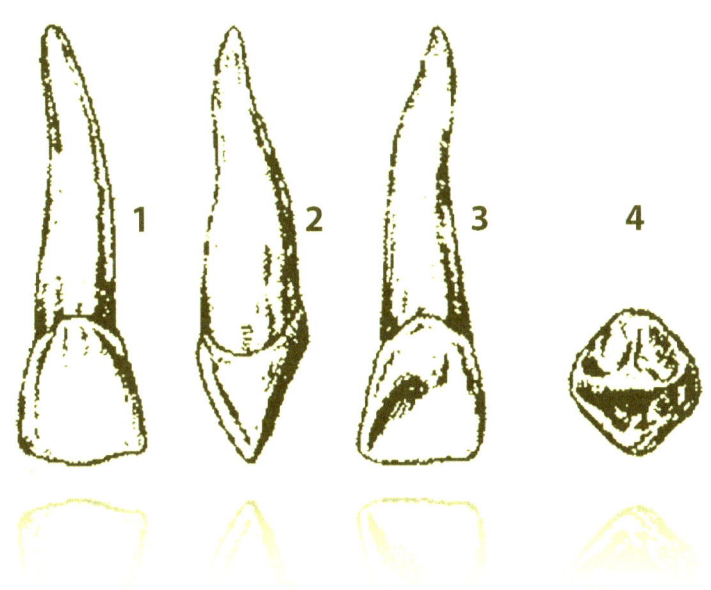

***Fig. 48 Milk incisor, medial,
and the lower (right) 584 917 219 498:***

1 – vestibular surface 514 817 219 648
2 – mesial surface 491 318 598 641
3 – lingual surface 461 598 597 681
4 – cutting surface 364 891 989 641

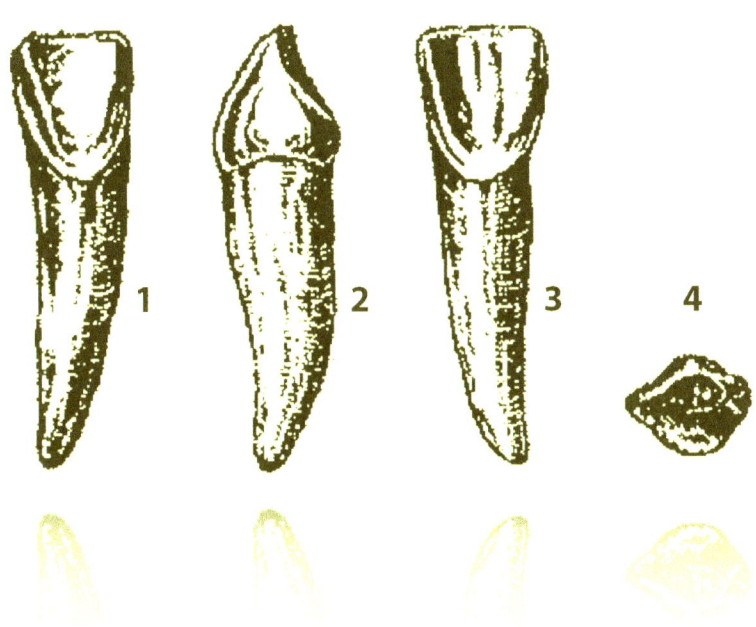

***Fig. 49 Milk incisor, lateral, bottom (right) 549 817 219 491:***
1 – vestibular surface 589 314 898 614
2 – mesial surface 386 149 948 511
3 – lingual surface 064 018 549 898
4 – cutting surface 414 818 619 710

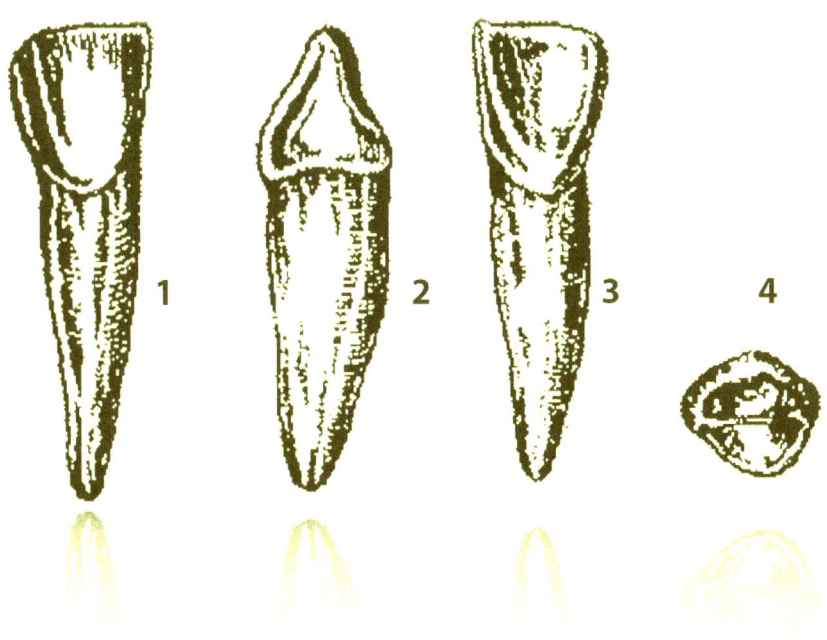

*Fig. 50 Milk canine, upper (right) 498 691 798 541:*
1 – vestibular surface 461 318 518 491
2 – mesial surface 498 641 319 814
3 – lingual surface 467 891 218 541
4 – cutting surface 318 491 819 617

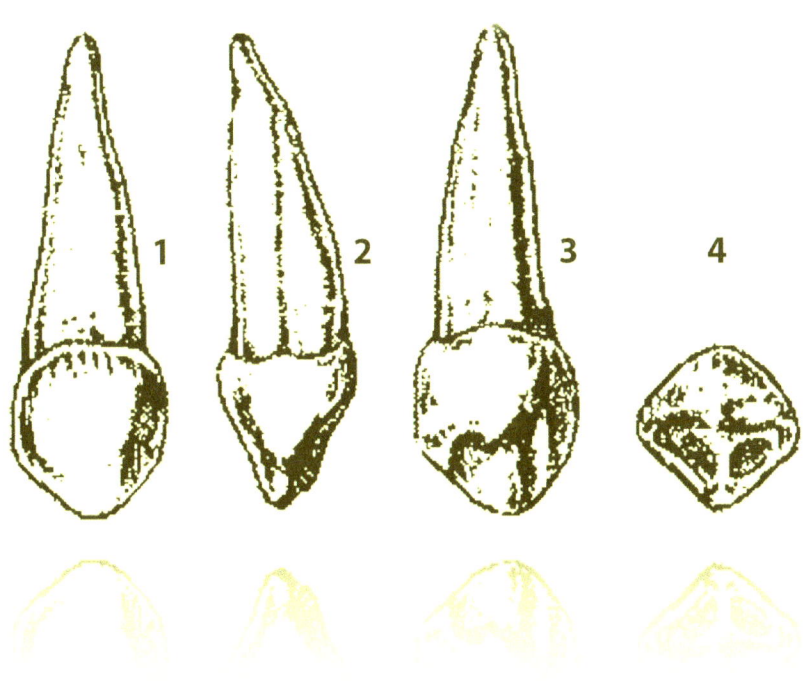

***Fig. 51 Milk canine, the lower (right) 619 317 218 491:***
1 – vestibular surface 218 491 319 614
2 – mesial surface 214 817 218 316
3 – lingual surface 648 517 219 491
4 – cutting surface 314 817 219 617

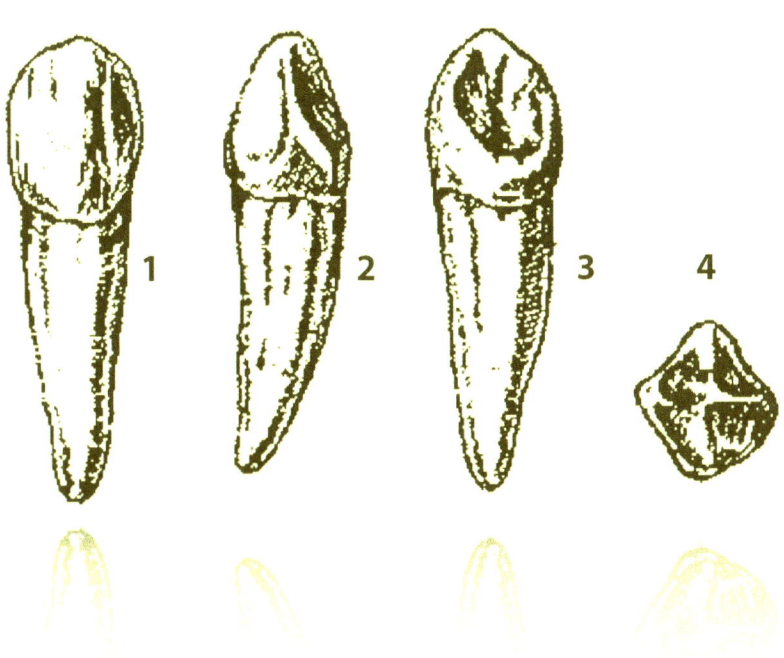

***Fig. 52 First molars, the first, the upper (right):***
1 – vestibular surface 491 718 519 497
2 – mesial surface 519 491 619 819
3 – lingual surface 594 817 219 648
4 – chewing surface 948 218 319 681

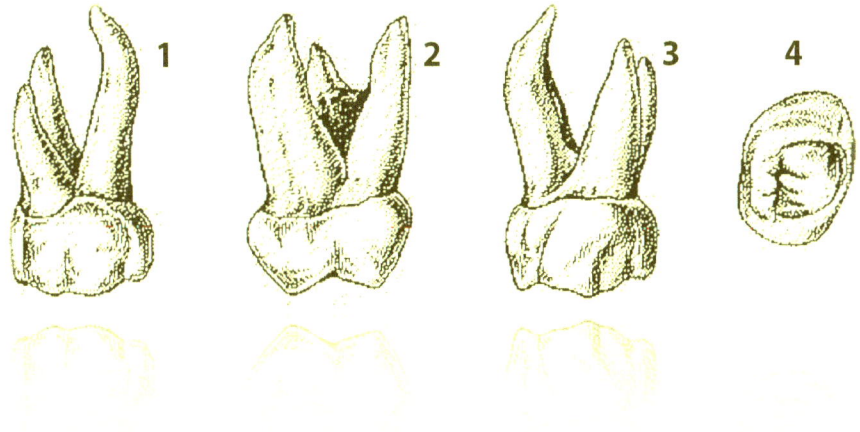

*Fig. 53 Molars, the second, the upper (right) 594 168 319 491:*
1 – vestibular surface 619 518 219 491
2 – mesial surface 469 518 319 641
3 – lingual surface 584 316 589 491
4 – chewing surface 891 498 319 617

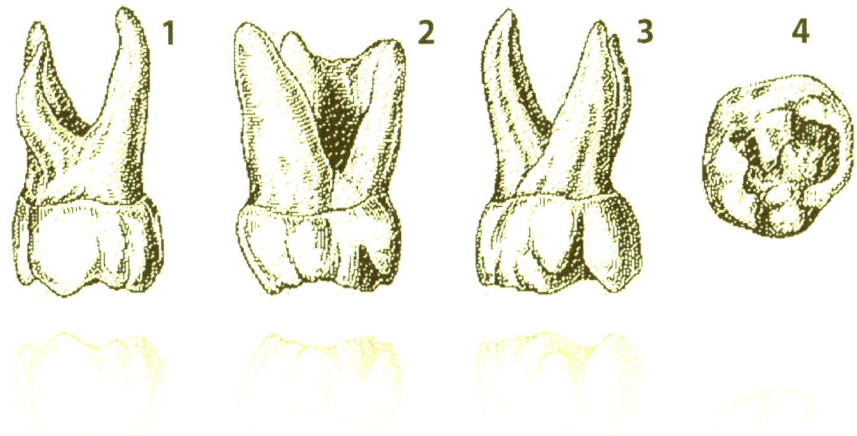

*Fig. 54 First molars, the lower (right) 491 318 519 491:*
1 – vestibular surface 614 817 219 817
2 – mesial surface 486 519 719 491
3 – lingual surface 801 698 598 641
4 – chewing surface 894 219 319 810

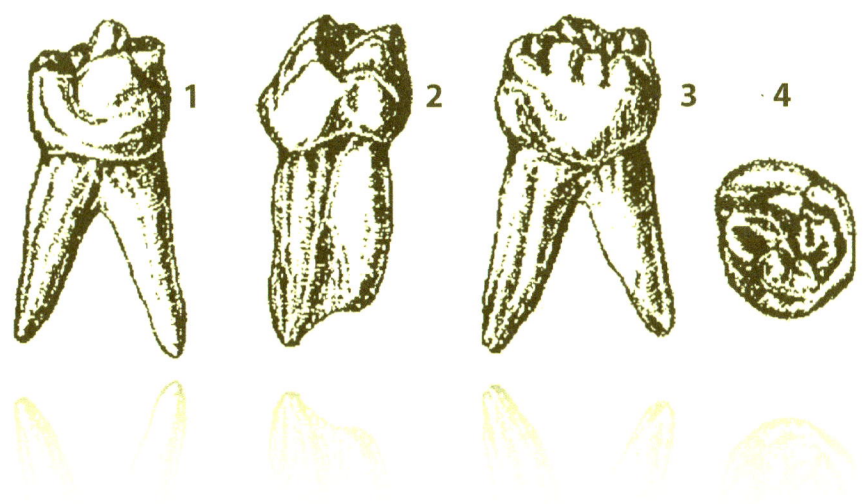

*Fig. 55 Second molars, the lower (right) 916 849 319 496:*
1 – vestibular surface 514 217 218 494
2 – mesial surface 584 564 819 718
3 – lingual surface 496 549 891 548
4 – chewing surface 649 817 918 491

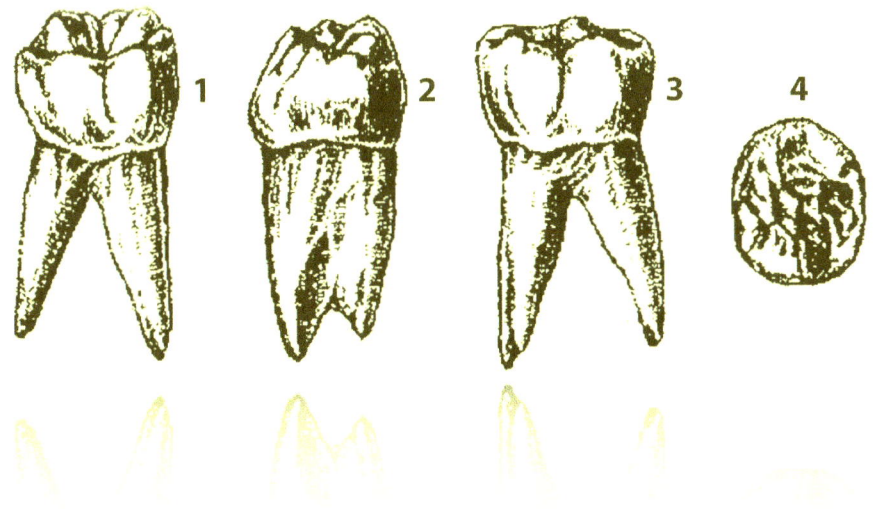

## Organs of oral cavity

### *Fig. 56 Lip 498 718 494 814:*

1 – the inner side of the lip (mouth cavity) 496 849 316 714
2 – submucosa 498 516 219 314
3 – mucous membrane 589 641 218 549
4 – Vermilion 598 714 219 674
5 – labial artery 598 541 219 491
6 – the circular muscle of mouth 548 321 818 221
7 – epidermis 598 718 889 888
8 – subcutaneous fat 594 817 549 164
9 – taste glands 198 016 219 491
10 – salivary glands 584 106 294 647
11 – the external side the lip (skin) 319 891 498 647

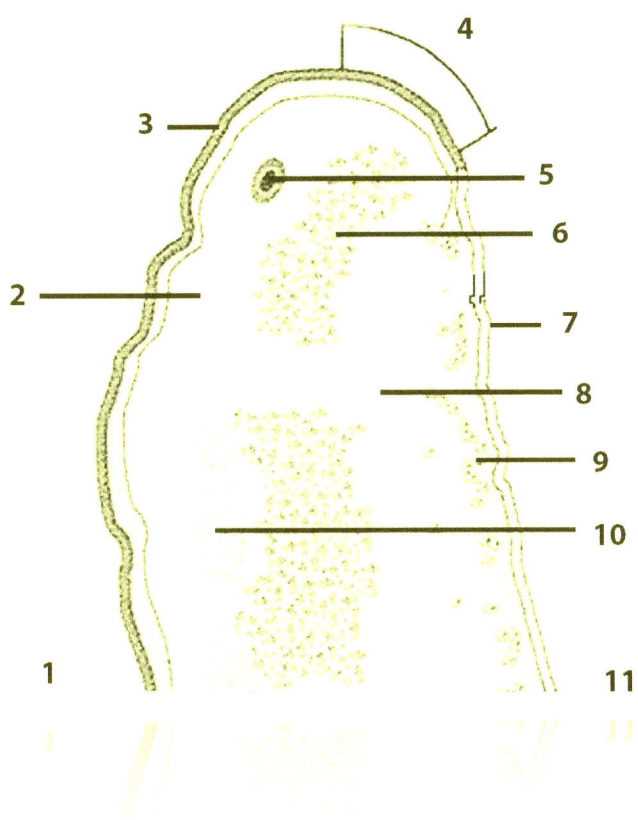

© Грабовой Г.П. 2002 127

*Fig. 57 Oral cavity and pharynx 489 461 319 891:*

1 – upper dental arch 514 618 519 714
2 – palatine raphe 318 549 219 641
3 – velopharyngeal arch 549 174 819 714
4 – palatine tonsil 514 218 319 671
5 – palato-lingual arch 479 604 594 219
6 – dorsum of tongue 489 617 218 481
7 – inferior dental arch 518 317 219 416
8 – lower lip 549 618 317 491
9 – pharynx 584 317 894 517
10 – commissure of lips 584 316 318 497
11 – tab (palatal) 314 841 219 647
12 – soft palate 549 561 718 649
13 – hard palate 564 817 219 481
14 – upper lip 314 816 319 471
15 – tubercle of the upper lip 648 716 498 721
16 – philtrum 642 148 894 216

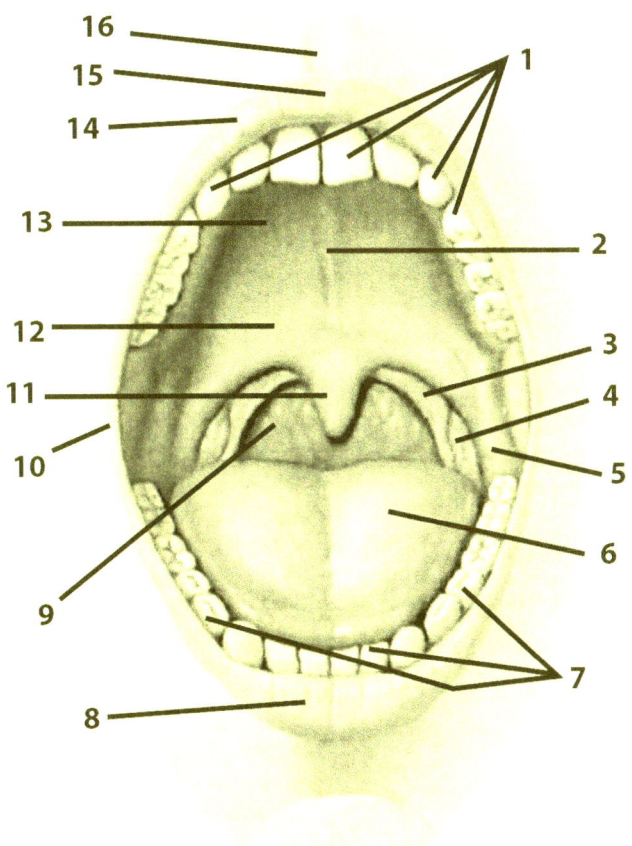

*Fig. 58 The mouth cavity 498 641 918 974 (Front. Tongue raised. Matter under the mucous membrane):*

1 – frenulum of the upper lip 498 691 719 497
2 – the gum of the upper jaw 898 691 319 497
3 – anterior lingual gland 486 194 718 541
4 – lingual nerve 214 318 714 818
5 – lower longitudinal muscle (of the tongue) 319 648 319 781
6 – tongue-tie 316 584 219 671
7 – the sublingual gland 849 671 219 371
8 – submandibular duct 896 318 316 948
9 – mandibular gum 519 318 219 641
10 – frenulum of the lower lip 318 364 891 871
11 – sublingual papilla 894 217 248 564
12 – bottom (diaphragm) of the mouth 548 612 016 498
13 – sublingual fold 421 649 198 791
14 – hypoglossis 219 064 284 714
15 – fimbriated fold 891 316 219 714

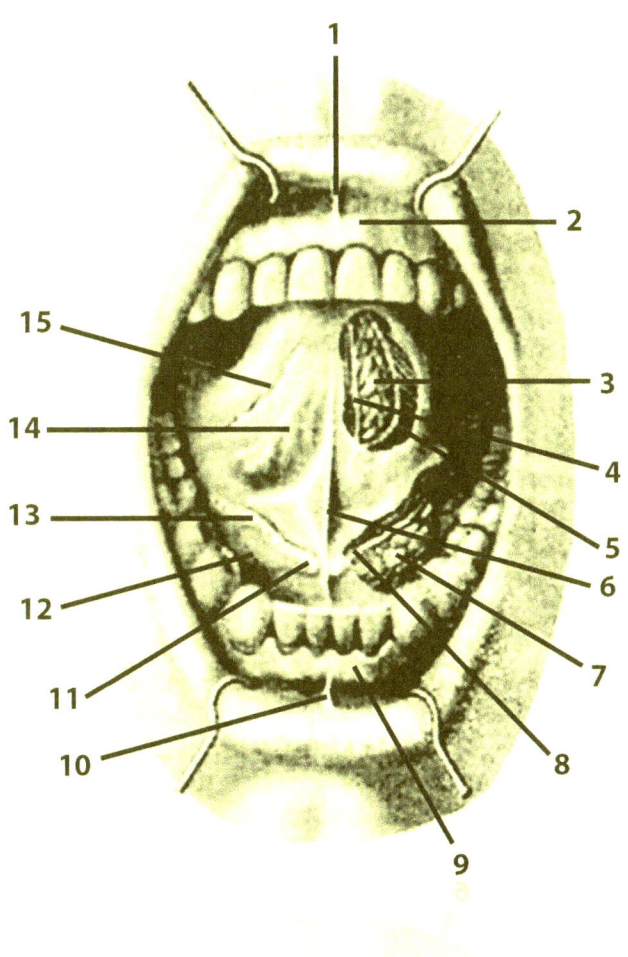

*Fig. 59 Tongue 398 716 219 841:*

1 – palatine tonsil 514 218 319 671
2 – lingual tonsil 498 791 648 219
3 – foliate papillae 418 644 319 515
4 – filiform papillae 589 617 298 471
5 – circumvallate papillae 891 319 481 617
6 – fungiform papillae 314 218 914 888

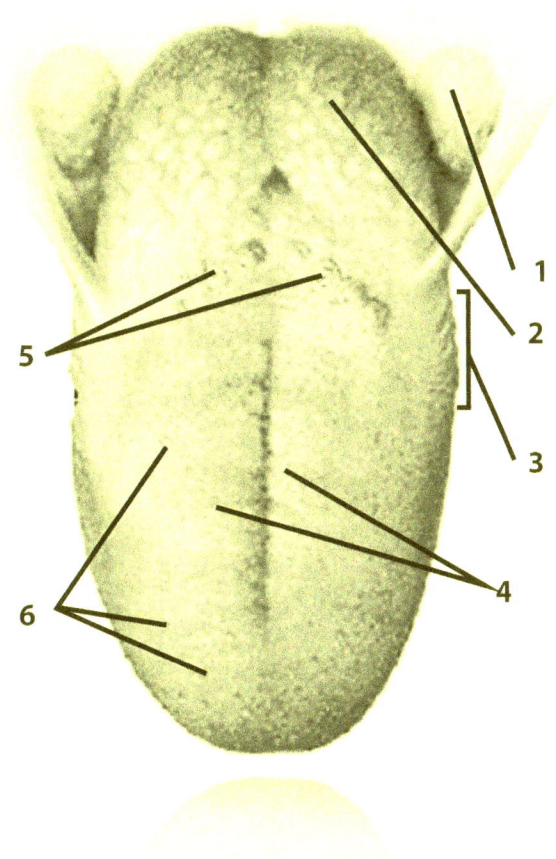

# Chewing and facial muscles

*Fig. 60 Muscles of tongue 594 218 598 641 (View on the right. Matter behind the right half of the upper and lower jaw):*

1 – palatoglossus muscle 194 891 319 491
2 – soft palate 549 561 718 649
3 – tongue 398 716 219 841
4 – hard palate 564 817 219 481
5 – lower jaw (part of image) 514 712 814 312
6 – genioglossal muscle 218 614 319 718
7 – inferior longitudinal muscle (of the tongue) 319 648 319 781
8 – hyoid bone 549 316 219 841
9 – the median thyrohyoid ligament 598 617 219 641
10 – thyroid cartilage 549 891 364 218
11 – inferior constrictor of pharynx 584 216 234 271
12 – thyrohyoid membrane 584 691 219 478
13 – chondroglossus muscle 594 281 319 641
14 – hyo-lingual muscle 814 316 498 384
15 – middle constrictor of pharynx 548 314 894 851
16 – styloglossus muscle 584 391 314 891
17 – stylopharyngeal muscle 598 617 218 491
18 – stylohyoid ligament 584 217 278 061
19 – upper constrictor of pharynx 348 541 618 714

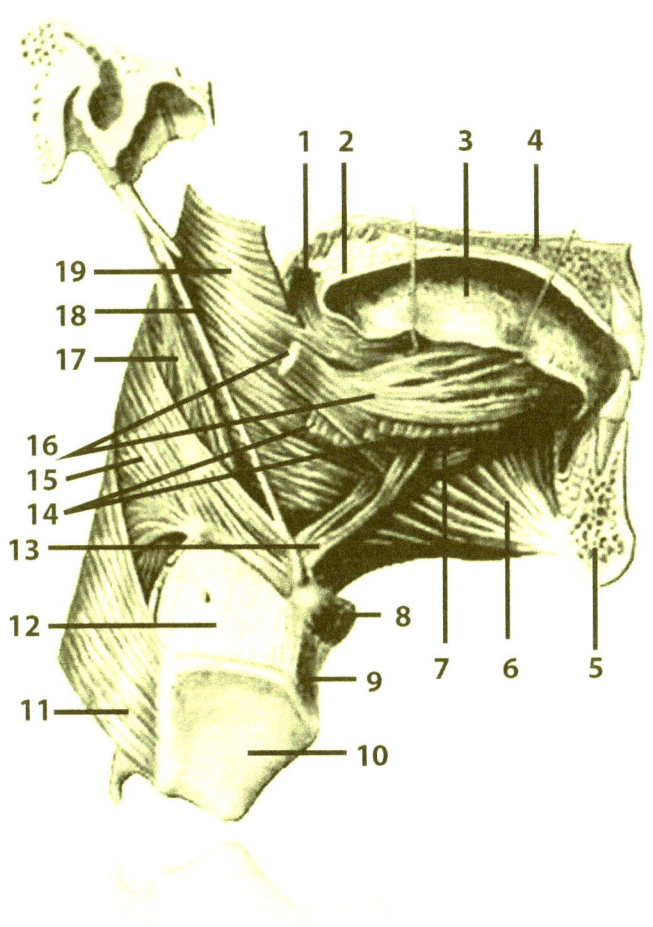

**Superficial facial muscles of head 219 317 914 817**
(Part 1 of Fig. 102)

**Facial muscles (front view) 598 641 398 719**
(Part 1 of Fig. 103)

**Deep facial muscles 328 721 428 919**
(Part 1 of Fig. 104)

**Chewing muscles 519 314 819 214**
(Part 1 of Fig. 105)

## Temporo-mandibular joint

***Fig. 61 Temporo-mandibular joint (sagittal view):***
1 – articular (condylar) process of the mandible 891 319 898 789
2 – head of the mandible 548 321 848 721
3 – joint capsule 498 641 718 491
4 – external auditory canal 519 421 919 811
5 – joint (intra-articular) disk 894 516 219 497
6 – mandibular fossa 558 912 918 222
7 – articular tubercle 288 412 298 322
8 – lateral pterygoid muscle 219 214 319 214
9 – temporal process of zygomatic bone 694 171 219 548
10 – coronoid process of the mandible 528 317 918 228

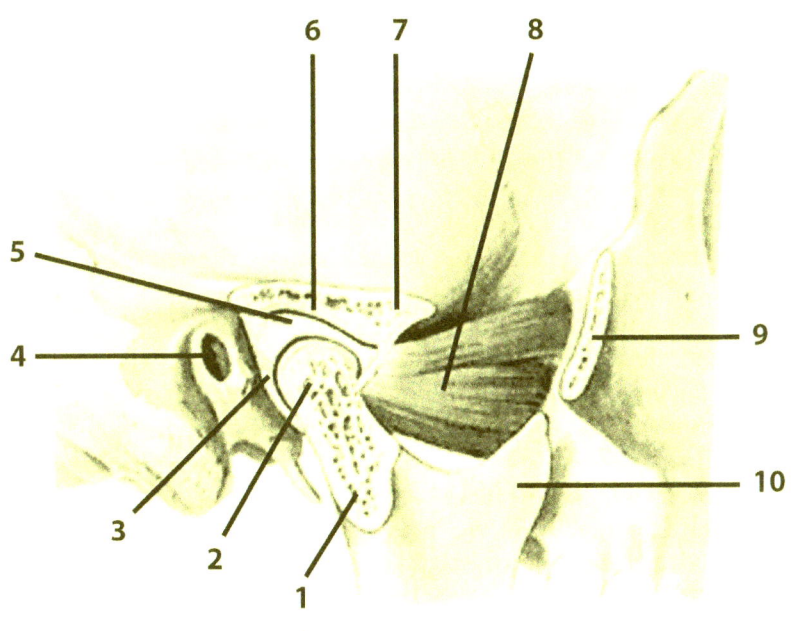

*Fig. 62 Bundles of temporomandibular joint
819 491 319 848 (view from the medial side):*

1 – lateral ligament (of temporomandibular joint) 519 647 218 541
2 – capsule of temporomandibular joint 498 641 718 491
3 – sphenomandibular ligament 584 317 219 497
4 – stylomandibular ligament 898 514 518 316
5 – opening of the lower jaw 489 201 319 871
6 – zygomatic arch 528 317 918 917
7 – sphenoid sinus 584 217 319 841
8 – pituitary fossa (sella turcica) 519 317 919 218

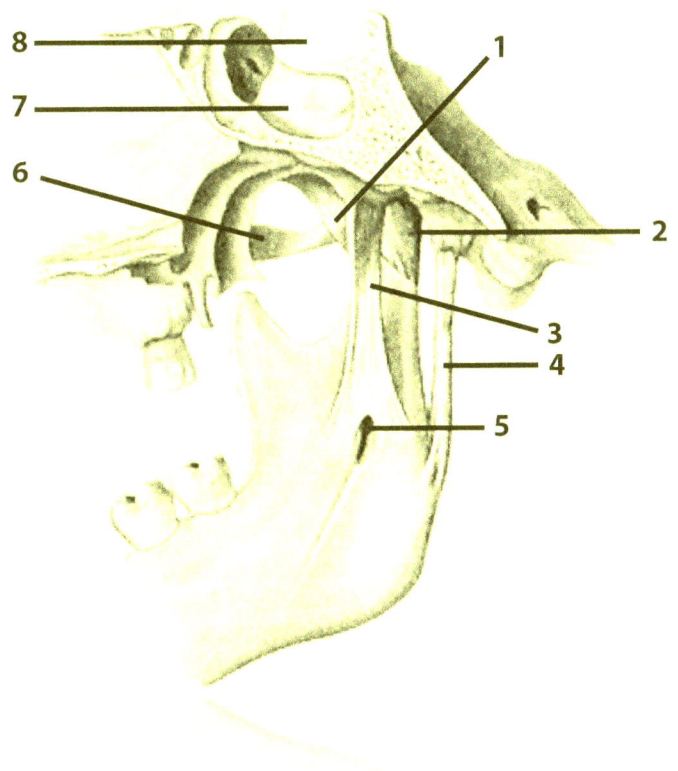

# Vestibular glands and oral cavity 498 617 219 491

*Fig. 63 Vestibular glands and oral cavity 498 617 219 491 (right side):*

1 – parotid gland 194 817 219 418

2 – parotid duct 218 491 619 317

3 – accessory parotid gland 514 816 719 497

4 – buccinator 549 317 849 217

5 – molar glands 514 817 219 498

6 – buccal glands 548 742 819 461

7 – labial glands 548 649 319 817

8 – upper lip 314 816 319 471

9 – tongue 398 716 219 841

10 – anterior lingual gland 486 194 718 541

11 – lower lip 549 618 317 491

12 – sublingual papilla 894 316 598 718

13 – large hypoglossal canal 548 717 219 418

14 – minor sublingual ducts 498 641 318 374

15 – mandible 514 712 814 312

16 – genioglossal muscle 218 614 319 718

17 – the sublingual gland 849 671 219 371

18 – mylohyoid muscle 498 541 316 841

19 – submandibular duct 896 318 316 948

20 – submandibular gland 498 714 319 481

21 – stylohyoid 594 217 298 647

22 – posterior belly of digastric muscle 316 849 918 716

23 – posterior lingual gland 314 849 216 371

24 – lower jaw 514 712 814 312

25 – masseter 598 712 918 212

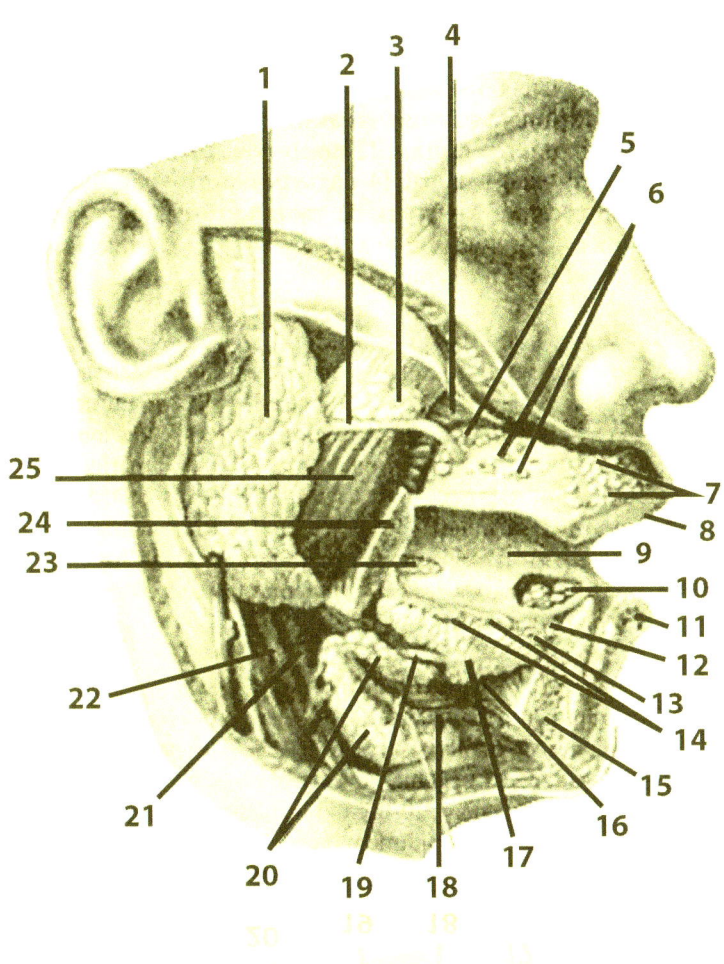

© Грабовой Г.П. 2002

# SPINE.
# CONNECTIONS, LIGAMENTS AND MUSCLES OF THE SPINE

## Spine 214 217 000 819
(Continue ) (Part 1 of Fig. 62)

***Fig. 64 Spine 214 217 000 819 (continued):***

A – physiological curves of the spine 598 614 818 017
primary curves 319 892 964 718
2 – thoracic kyphosis 379 491 814 219
4 – sacral kyphosis 598 061 719 898
secondary curves 598 718 419 061
1 – cervical lordosis 898 716 919 041
4 – lumbar lordosis 584 061 718 910
B – The spinal canal 521 314 818 214

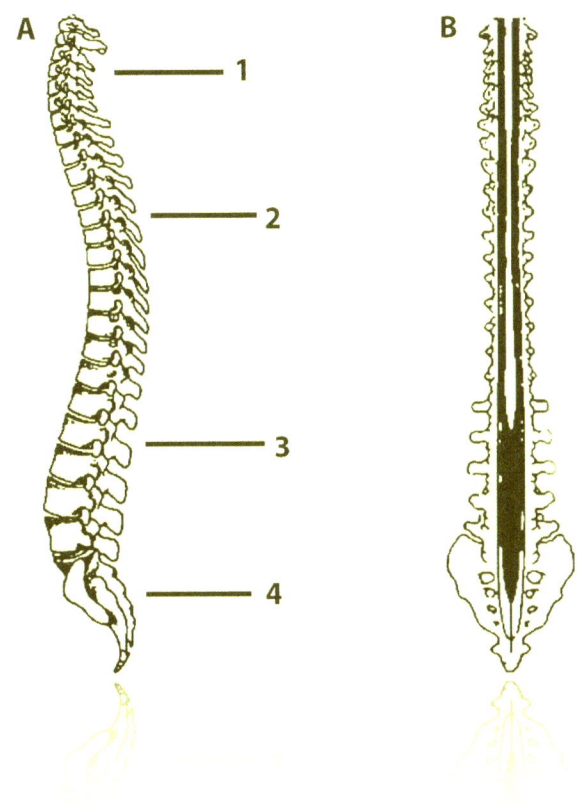

## Vertebrae 498 641 319 048

*Fig. 65 The first cervical vertebra (atlas) 914 816 978 496:*

A – top view
B – bottom view
1 – posterior tubercle 894 217 319 498
2 – posterior arch 894 617 319 497
3 – vertebral foramen 864 914 898 516
4 – groove for vertebral artery 749 891 218 641
5 – superior glenoid fossa 598 691 219 674
6 – lateral opening (foramen of the transverse process) 649 581 219 697
7 – transverse process 584 316 918 581
8 – lateral mass 648 719 218 541
9 – tooth pit 694 197 289 471
10 – anterior tubercle 319 691 218 712
11 – anterior arch 649 171 218 641
12 – inferior glenoid fossa 598 317 294 817

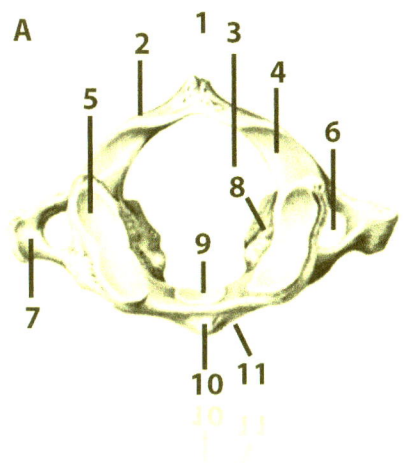

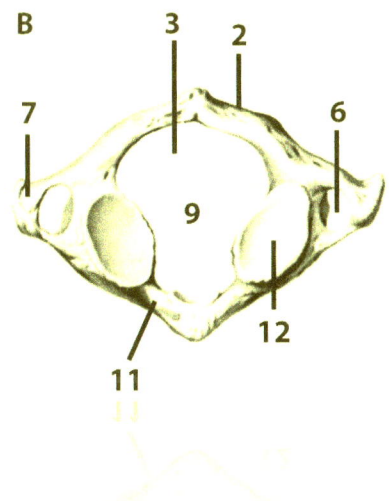

***Fig. 66 The second cervical vertebra (axis) 794 218 849 617:***

A – front view

B – side view

1 – dens of the axis 598 314 219 617

2 – anterior articular surface 698 591 219 491

3 – the vertebral body 598 674 218 514

4 – superior articular process 589 491 218 641

5 – transverse process 698 371 294 811

6 – lower articular process 541 319 894 361

7 – the vertebral arch 898 561 219 364

8 – spinous process 581 319 619 714

9 – posterior articular surface 598 612 819 498

10 – lateral opening (foramen of the transverse process) 594 612 898 714

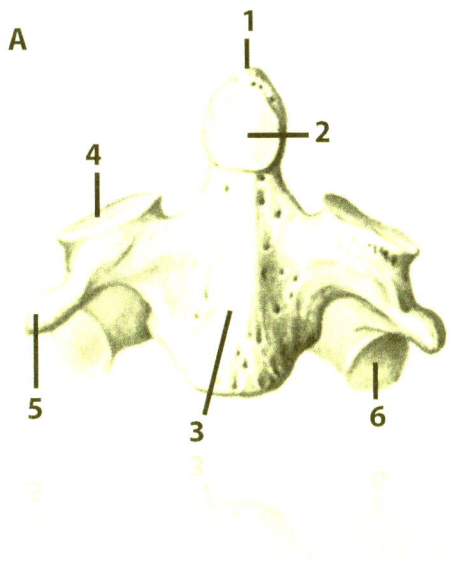

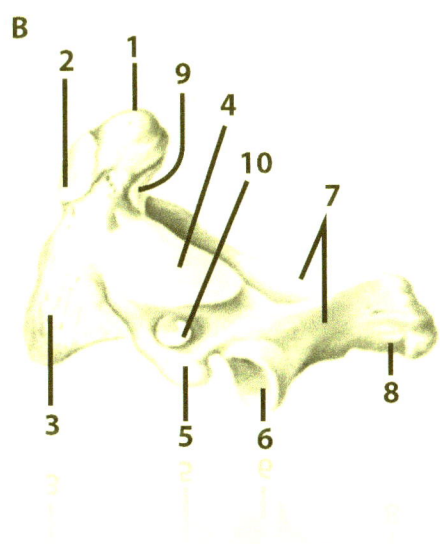

***Fig. 67 Cervical vertebra***
***(III - VI cervical vertebrae) 498 317 218 641:***

A – front view

B – top view

1 – spinous process 514 217 218 684

2 – vertebral foramen 319 648 281 317

3 – the vertebral arch 094 701 278 649

4 – superior articular process 894 361 219 897

5 – transverse process 698 317 298 641

6 – posterior tubercle of the transverse process 550 694 931 074

7 – anterior tubercle of the transverse process 894 171 219 647

8 – lateral opening (foramen of the transverse process) 589 316 298 649

9 – vertebral body 368 174 289 691

10 – inferior articular process 519 581 314 891

11 – groove for spinal nerve 649 718 219 417

12 – uncus corporis 689 517 219 618

13 – superior vertebral notch 216 541 319 714

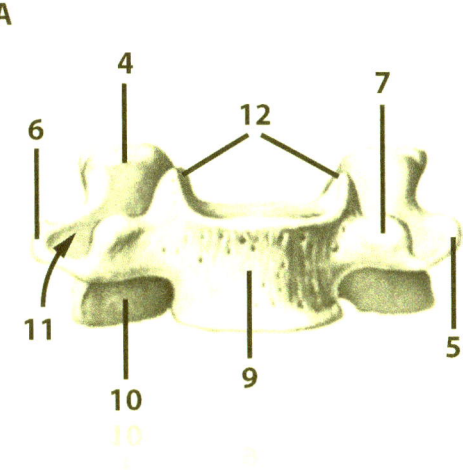

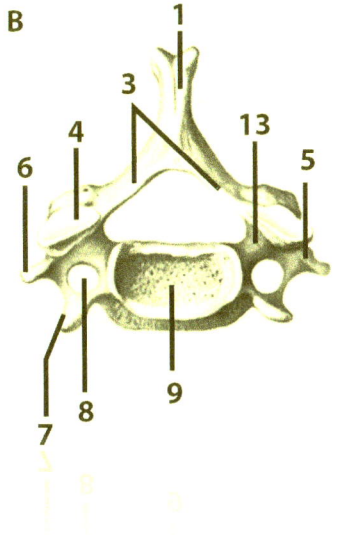

*Fig. 68 Seventh cervical vertebra 319 648 519 647:*

A – side view

B – top view

1 – superior articular process 584 216 549 617

2 – superior vertebral notch 594 691 798 714

3 – the vertebral body 918 694 319 896

4 – transverse process 698 712 319 641

5 – inferior vertebral notch 549 598 694 714

6 – inferior articular process 548 217 219 691

7 – spinous process 591 316 214 278

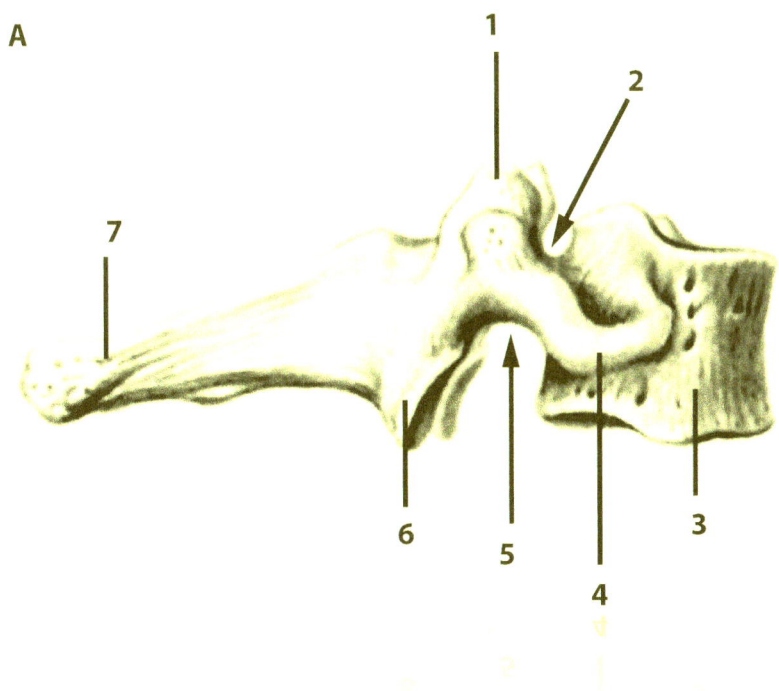

*Fig. 69 Thoracic vertebra 542 317 212 227:*

A – top view
B – side view
1 – spinous process 518 617 218 141
2 – the vertebral arch 648 549 819 712
3 – transverse process 598 642 319 811
4 – vertebral foramen 798 621 319 416
5 – pedicle of arch of vertebra 498 317 218 217
6 – the vertebral body 517 219 319 617
7 – superior costal fovea 549 312 814 212
8 – superior articular process 219 715 319 215
9 – transverse ribs fossa (rib fossa of the transverse process) 821 319 921 819
10 – plate of vertebral arch 514 218 619 719
11 – superior vertebral notch 598 641 398 011
12 – inferior rib fovea 019 712 219 312
13 – inferior vertebral notch 512 314 812 214
14 – inferior articular process 528 644 328 016

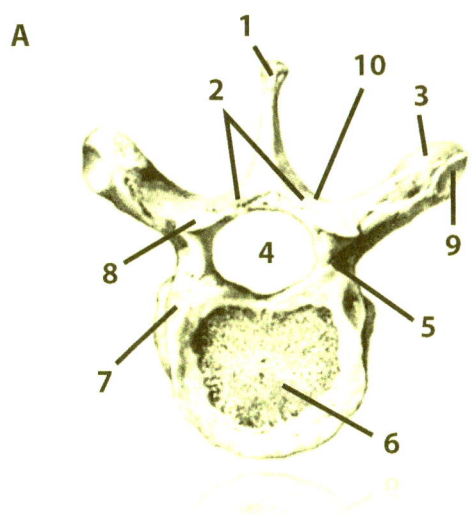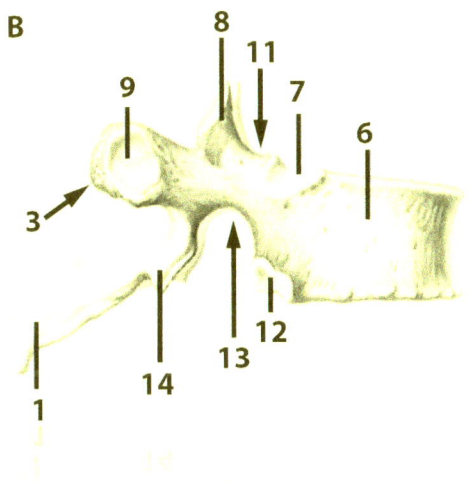

***Fig. 70 XII thoracic vertebra (XI and XII thoracic vertebrae) (side view) 496 819 318 514:***

1 – spinous process 314 815 619 718
2 – transverse process 218 316 514 471
3 – the vertebral body 364 819 519 614
4 – costal fovea 818 542 617 218
5 – superior articular process 514 618 019 008
6 – superior vertebral notch 194 691 298 511
7 – inferior vertebral notch 584 317 218 584
8 – inferior articular process 549 613 219 814
9 – accessory process 319 684 218 514
10 – mastoid process 819 617 218 419

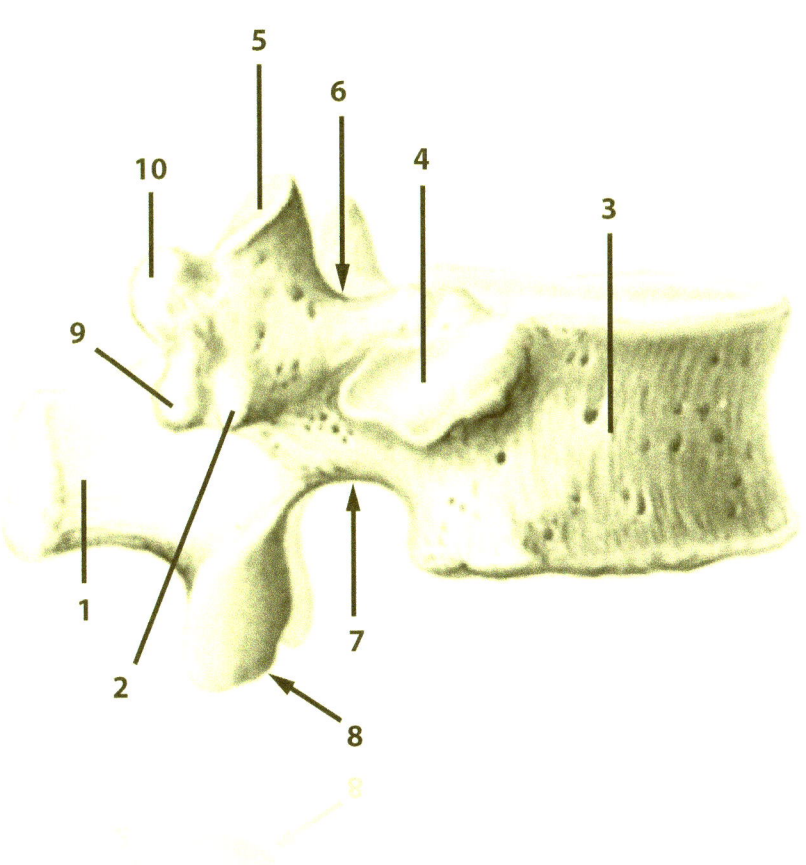

*Fig. 71 Lumbar vertebra 618 513 219 418:*

A – top view
B – side view
C – rear view
1 – spinous process 513 219 813 919
2 – vertebral arch 391 498 016 217
3 – inferior articular process 549 316 218 494
4 – superior articular process 519 617 299 017
5 – mastoid process 918 217 319 817
6 – accessory process 518 431 219 917
7 – costal process 317 814 214 917
8 – vertebral foramen 828 317 918 217
9 – pedicle of vertebral arch 498 317 218 217
10 – vertebral body 598 641 319 071
11 – superior vertebral notch 518 491 316 498
12 – inferior vertebral notch 549 617 219 811
13 – vertebral foramen (the projection of foramen) 828 317 918 217

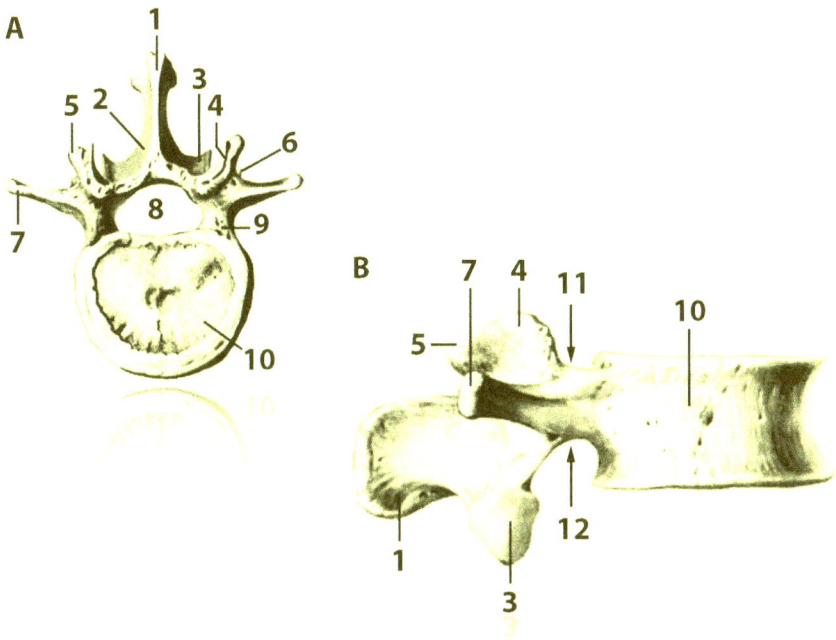
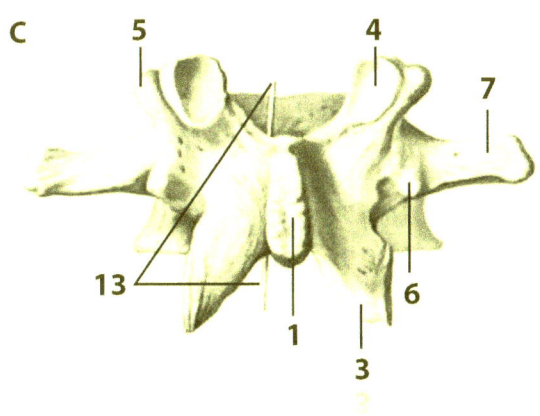

© Грабовой Г.П. 2002

***Fig. 72 Sacrum 514 716 814 226***
*(front view, pelvic surface):*

1 – base of sacrum 519 614 319 812
2 – superior articular process 519 328 919 228
3 – lateral part 319 712 919 212
4 – transverse lines 428 213 328 333
5 – anterior sacral foramen 489 213 217 289
6 – top of the sacrum 408 217 229 327
7 – sacral wing 519 618 514 217
8 – sacral vertebrae 584 317 218 498

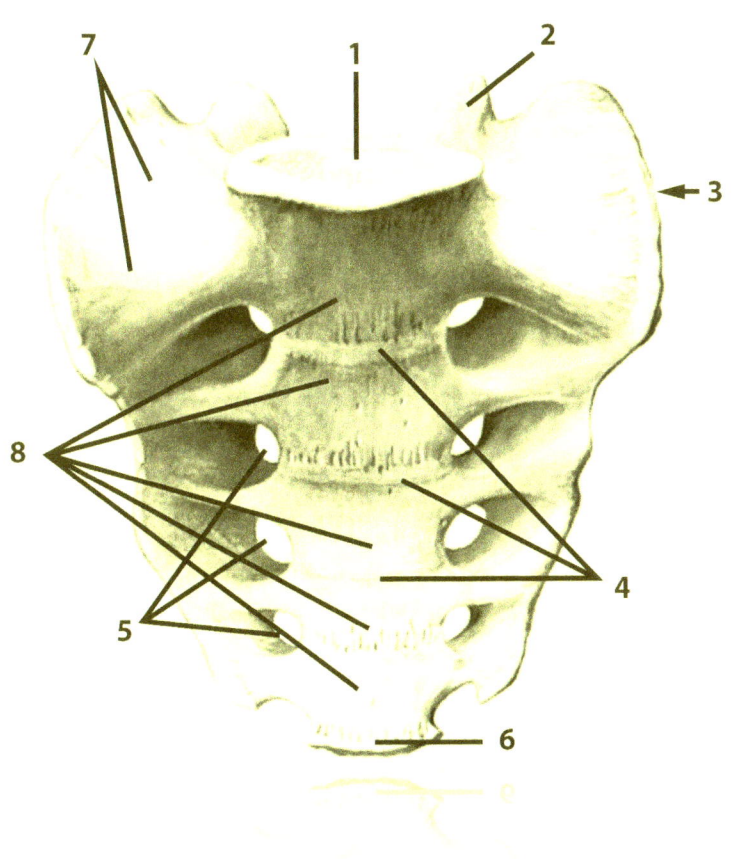

***Fig. 73 sacrum 514 716 814 226:***

A – rear view (dorsal surface)

B – side view

C – inner-view of the mid-longitudinal plane

1 – sacral canal (superior foramen) 594 647 289 391

2 – superior articular process 519 328 919 228

3 – sacral tuberosity 498 316 219 471

4 – auriculate surface 594 561 378 541

5 – lateral sacral crest 584 816 219 471

6 – intermediate sacral crest 319 641 281 491

7 – sacral hiatus (the inferior opening of sacral canal) 316 218 319 091

8 – sacral horns 019 001 849 471

9 – dorsal (posterior) sacral foramina 698 041 278 914

10 – the median sacral crest 518 691 298 741

11 – base of sacrum 519 614 319 812

12 – apex of the sacrum 408 217 229 327

13 – sacral canal 584 621 319 647

14 – anterior sacral foramen 489 213 217 289

15 – intervertebral foramen 584 101 294 988

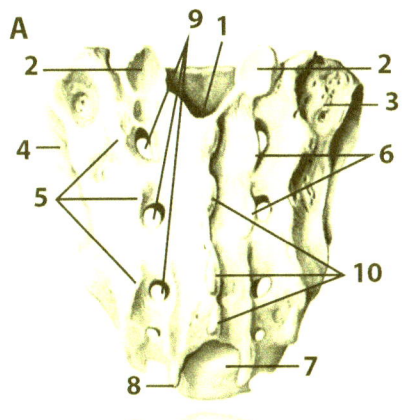
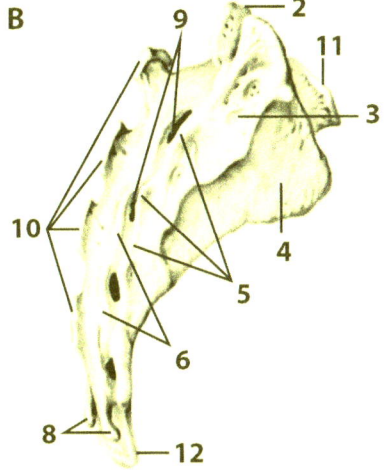
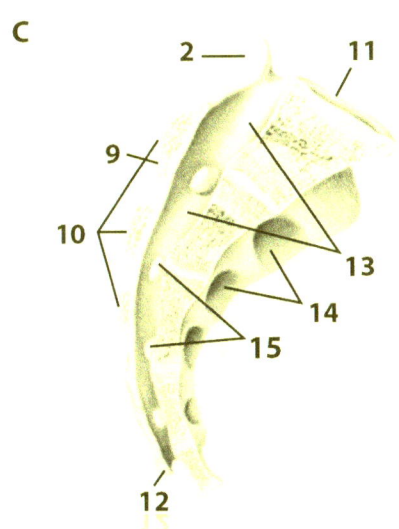

© Грабовой Г.П. 2002 165

**Pelvis 584 316 719 041**

**Pelvic bone (right) (view from the lateral side)
214 317 918 227 (Part 1, Fig. 89A)**

**Pelvic bone (right) (view from the medial side)
214 317 918 227 (Part 1, Fig. 89B)**

**Coccyx 519 513 819 213 (Part 1, Fig. 59)**

© Грабовой Г.П. 2002

**Spinal motor segment 714 986 219 694**

*Fig. 74 Spinal motor segment 714 986 219 694:*
1 – nerve root 519 691 219 814
2 – spinal cord 314 218 814 719
3 – the intervertebral foramen 517 218 916 284
4 – intervertebral disc 648 217 398 491
5 – the vertebral body 849 161 219 711

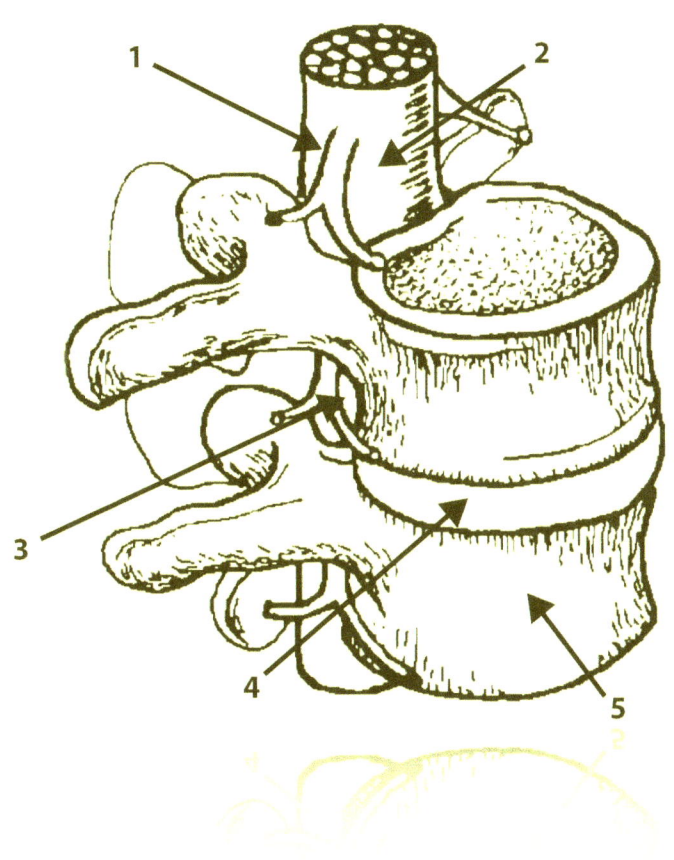

© Грабовой Г.П. 2002

**Muscles and ligaments of the spine 549 641 894 217**
Compounds of the spine 894 216 819 048
Syndesmosis (ligaments) of spinal column 398 947 019 818
Synchondrosis of spinal column 519 312 498 061
Spinal column joints 719 891 498 061

***Fig. 75 Junctions of vertebrae (sagittal projection at the level of two lumbar vertebrae) 498 641 917 218:***

A – intervertebral symphysis 898 064 317 219

B – zygapophysial joint 598 071 319 481

1 – vertebral body 598 641 319 071

2 – nucleus pulposus of the intervertebral disc 514 891 518 316

3 – anterior longitudinal ligament 689 174 219 814

4 – the fibrous ring of the intervertebral disk 498 716 219 714

5 – superior articular process of the lumbar vertebrae 519 617 299 017

6 – posterior longitudinal ligament 548 691 218 781

7 – the intervertebral foramen of the lumbar spine 916 048 219 491

8 – yellow ligament 549 488 194 016

9 – joint capsule of zygapophysial (intervertebral) joint 364 198 278 471

10 – interspinous ligament 368 142 894 216

11 – supraspinal ligament 890 149 540 691

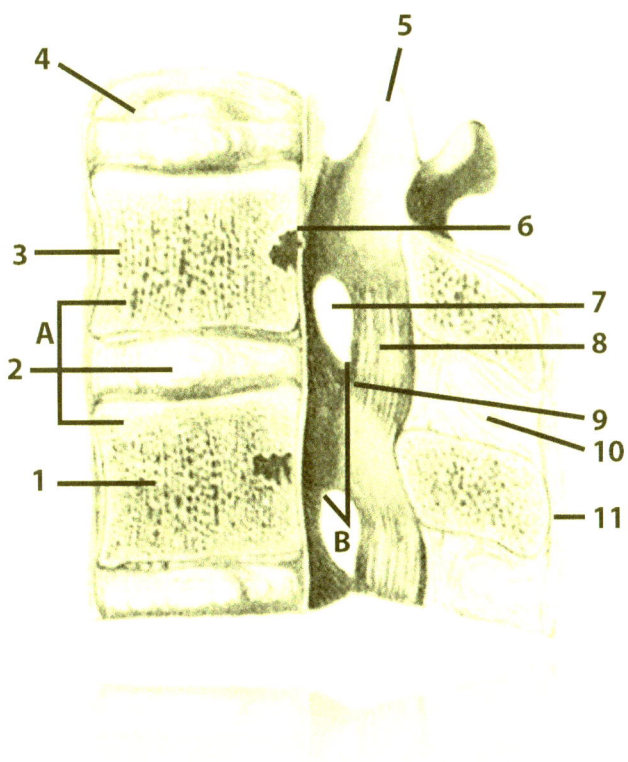

*Fig. 76 The junctions between the occipital bone and the I-II cervical vertebrae 379 814 919 718:*

1 – transverse ligament of the first cervical vertebra 589 061 319 498
2 – occipital bone 214 712 219 312
3 – Atlanto-occipital joint 591 048 319 491
4 – I cervical vertebra 914 816 978 496
5 – cruciate ligament of atlas 618 717 919 064
6 – II cervical vertebra 794 218 849 617
7 – pterygoid ligament 598 019 318 941
8 – longitudinal beams 541 061 719 801
9 – tectorial membrane 391 848 319 064
10 – ligament of the tooth apex 718 391 898 491
11 – dens of the axis 598 314 219 617
12 – clivus of the skull base 319 778 219 228
13 – lateral atlantoaxial joint 719 891 906 217
14 – middle atlantoaxial joint 598 089 319 641
15 – glenoid cavity of the middle atlantoaxial joint 489 061 918 217
16 – posterior longitudinal ligament 384 619 818 061

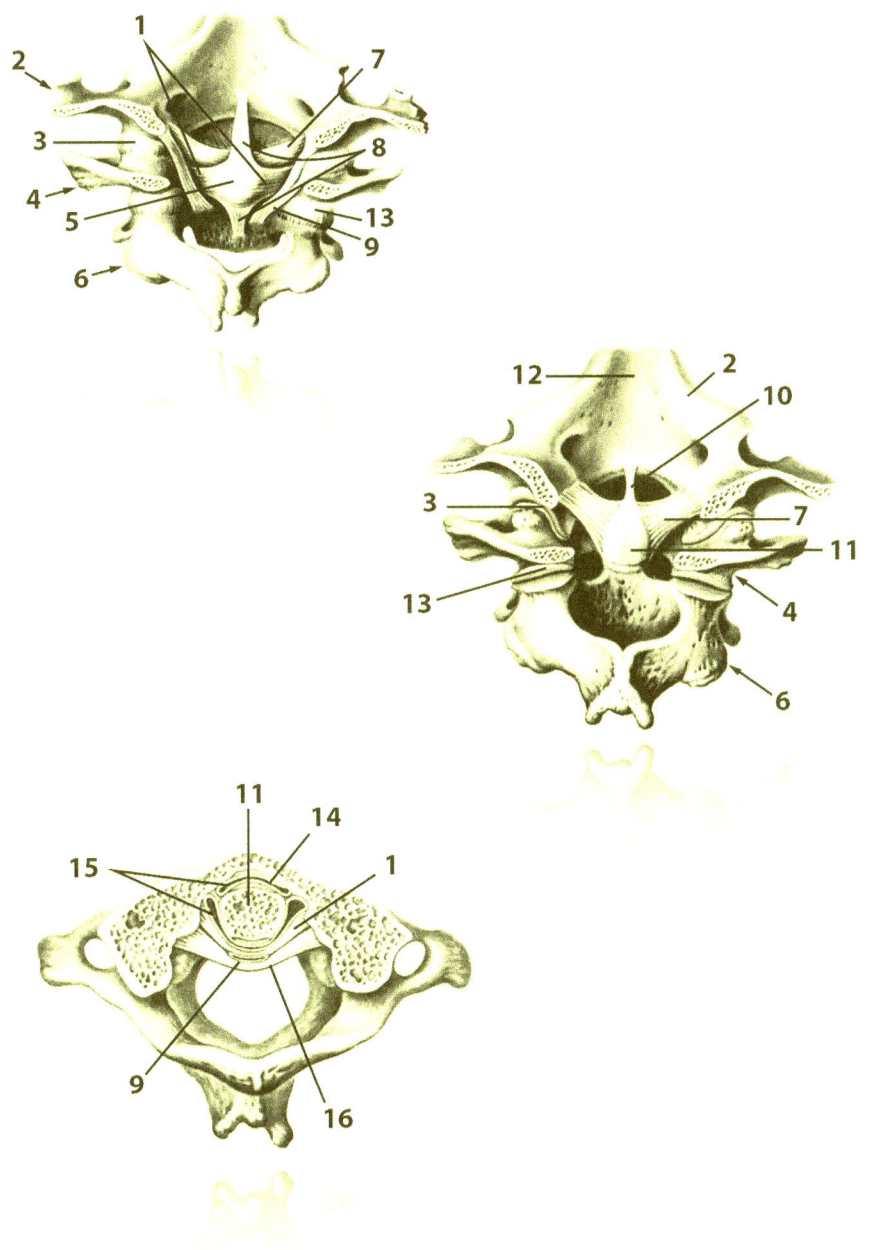

© Грабовой Г.П. 2002

*Fig. 77 Ligaments of the cervical vertebrae and occipital bone 718 119 498 064:*

1 – posterior occipital membrane 598 817 319 048
2 – nuchal ligament 517 319 049 811
3 – anterior occipital ligament 490 391 849 061
4 – anterior occipital membrane 598 601 819 317
5 – I cervical vertebra 914 816 978 496
6 – lateral atlantoaxial joint 719 891 906 217
7 – occipital bone 214 712 219 312
8 – lateral occipital ligament 974 217 298 041
9 – II cervical vertebra 794 218 849 617
10 – yellow ligament 549 488 194 016

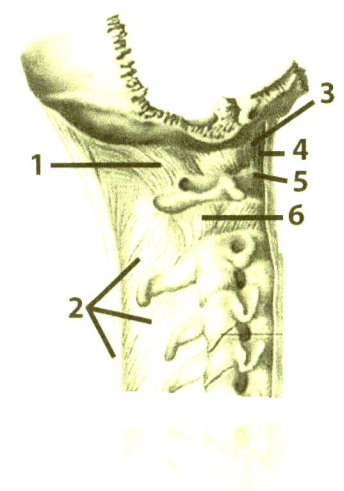

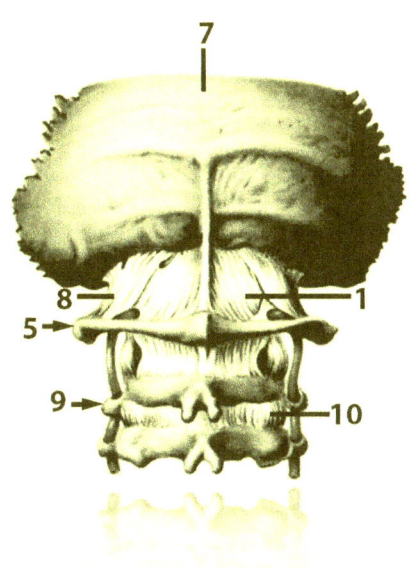

© Грабовой Г.П. 2002

*Fig. 78 Ligaments of the spine (thoracic region) costovertebral joints 514 891 219 478:*

1 – ligament of rib tubercle 698 714 219 811
2 – supraspinal ligament 890 149 540 691
3 – yellow ligament 549 488 194 016
4 – costo-transverse ligament 948 691 219 794
5 – lateral costotransverse ligament 894 691 217 474
6 – intertransverse ligaments 514 692 899 714
7 – internal intercostal membrane 598 726 319 491

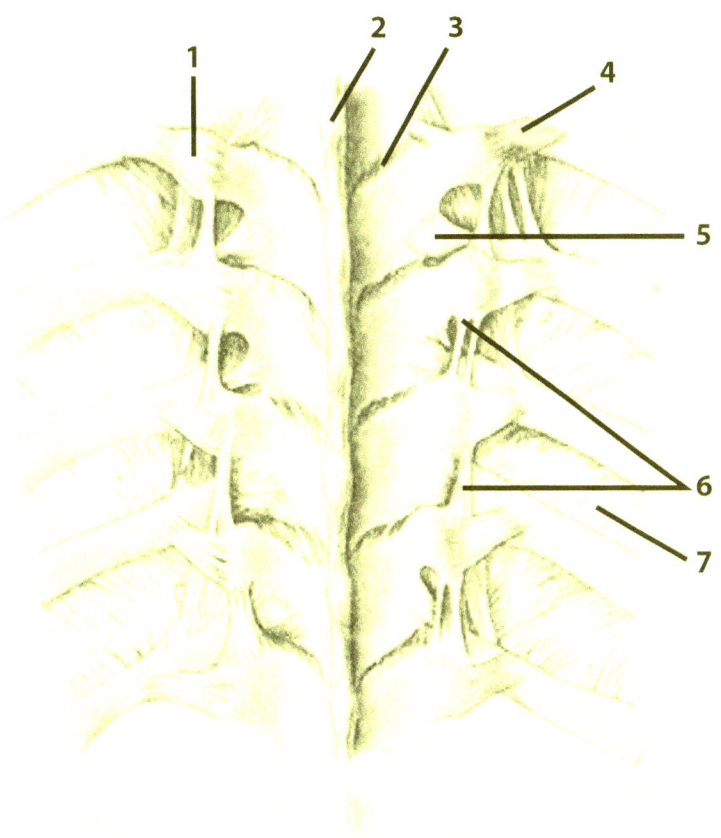

***Fig. 79 intervertebral disc 648 217 398 491:***
1 – Pulposus (gelatinous) kernel 514 891 518 316
2 – fibrous ring 498 716 219 714

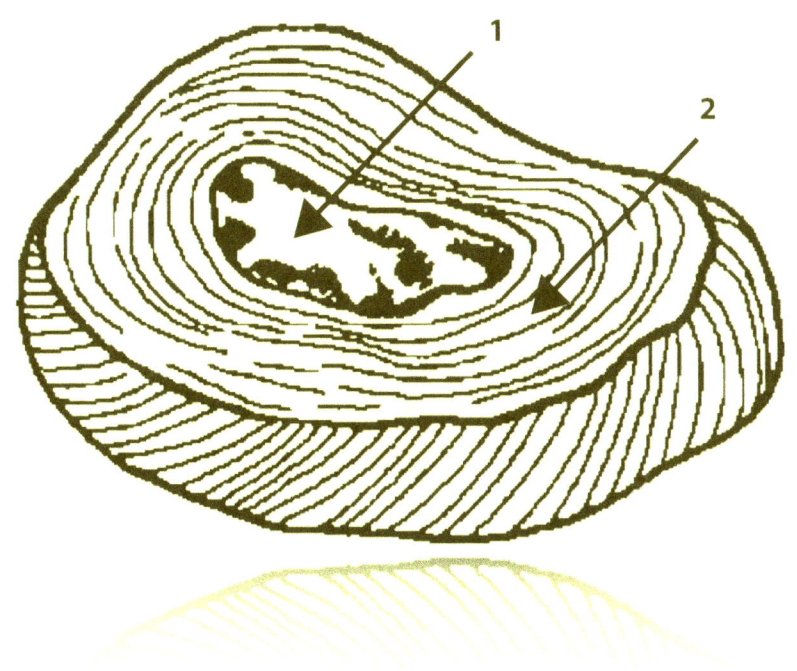

# Ligaments of the pelvis and hip joint 498 641 798 478

*Fig. 80 Ligaments of the pelvis and hip joint 498 641 798 478:*
A – Front View
1 – IV lumbar vertebra 467 198 219 481
2 – anterior longitudinal ligament 848 471 219 819
3 – iliolumbar ligament 319 641 289 798
4 – inguinal ligament 949 641 289 541
5 – articular capsule of the hip joint 589 671 218 498
6 – iliac-femoral ligament 364 911 894 564
7 – obturator membrane 312 689 319 716
8 – pubic symphysis 368 214 598 471
9 – pubic arcuate ligament 496 549 718 614
10 – superior pubic ligament 894 216 218 498
11 – greater trochanter 519 814 089 319
12 – anterior superior iliac spine 379 041 298 517
13 – ventral sacroiliac ligament 589 491 291 478
14 – lumbosacral joint 591 071 298 498
15 – anterior sacrococcygeal ligament 578 601 949 011

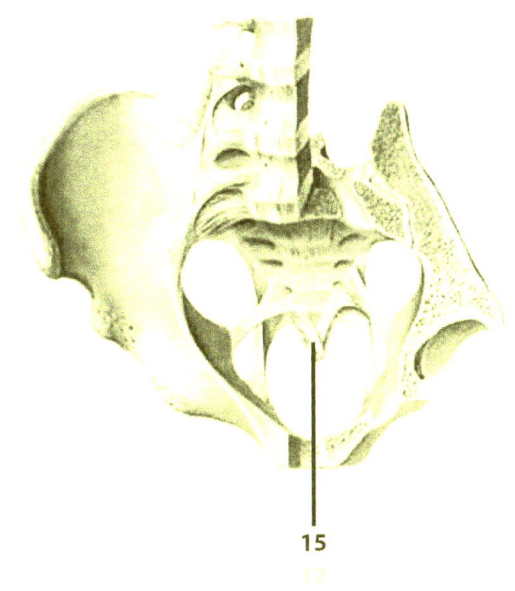

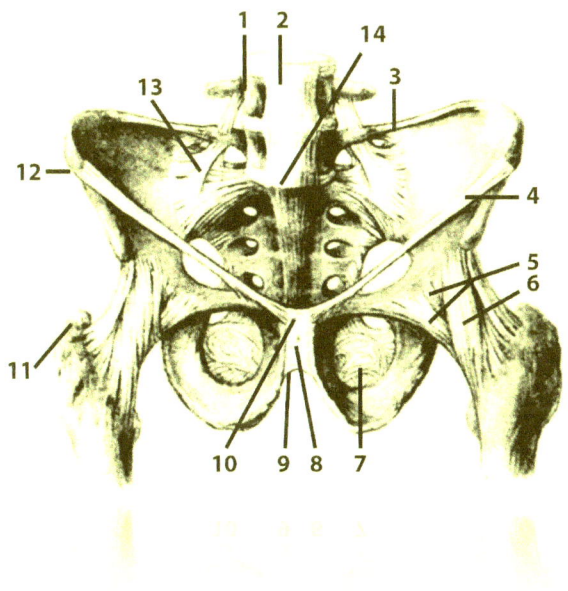

© Грабовой Г.П. 2002

*Fig. 80 Ligaments of the pelvis and hip joint 498 641 798 478:*
B – rear view
1 – iliolumbar ligament 479 681 598 718
2 – dorsal sacroiliac ligament 574 981 319 818
3 – superficial dorsal sacrococcygeal ligament 498 688 715 301
4 – deep dorsal sacrococcygeal ligament 594 072 319 401
5 – dorsal lateral sacrococcygeal ligament 719 317 908 481
6 – sacrotuberal ligament 501 489 714 211
7 – sacrococcygeal joint 291 081 407 201

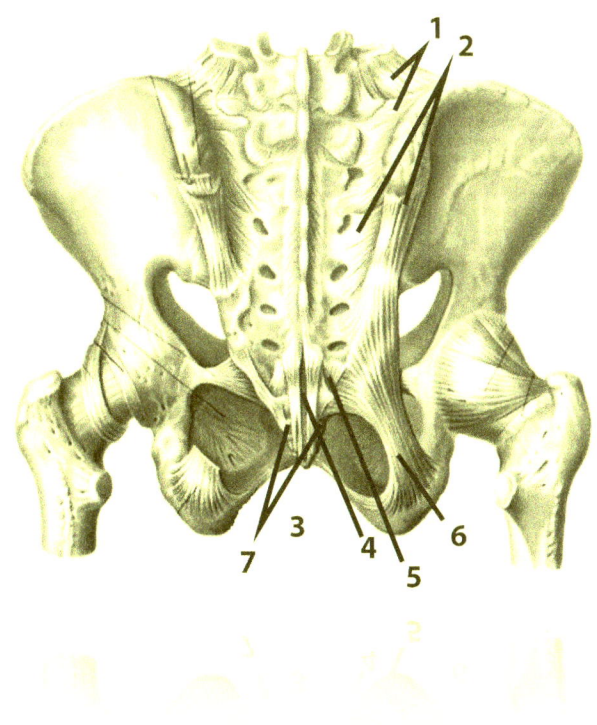

© Грабовой Г.П. 2002

# MUSCLES AND FASCIA OF BACK AND NECK 798 041 261 509

## Superficial muscles of the back 819 314 914 812

(Part 1 of Fig. 97)

*Fig. 81 Muscles of the back and the rear part of the neck (superficial muscles, first second and third layers) 519 648 218 741:*

1 – semispinal muscle of head 914 217 218 498
2 – Belt muscle of head 298 742 279 488
3 – Belt muscle of neck 216 498 948 741
4 – muscle lifting the shoulder blade 214 317 914 717
5 – small rhomboid muscle 319 061 919 618
6 – greater rhomboid muscle 584 317 914 016
7 – supraspinatus muscle 312 214 812 514
8 – infraspinatus muscle (partial view) 894 314 818 574
9 – minor circular muscle (part of image) 498 518 491 748
10 – greater circular muscle (part of image) 849 516 319 478
11 – latissimus dorsi muscle 429 318 829 998
12 – aponeurosis of the latissimus dorsi muscle 549 718 219 478
13 – external oblique muscle of abdomen 529 312 419 272
14 – lumbar triangle 894 568 514 811
15 – gluteal fascia 598 314 698 718
16 – middle gluteus muscle 589 491 219 641
17 – minor gluteus muscle 364 917 584 218
18 – piriform muscle 498 571 218 498
19 – superior gemellus muscle 364 581 219 644
20 – obturator internus muscle 398 711 264 814
21 – inferior gemellus muscle 314 894 219 471
22 – gluteus maximus muscle (part of image) 548 361 894 317
23 – square thigh muscle 694 584 219 471
24 – ischial tuberosity 529 312 918 812

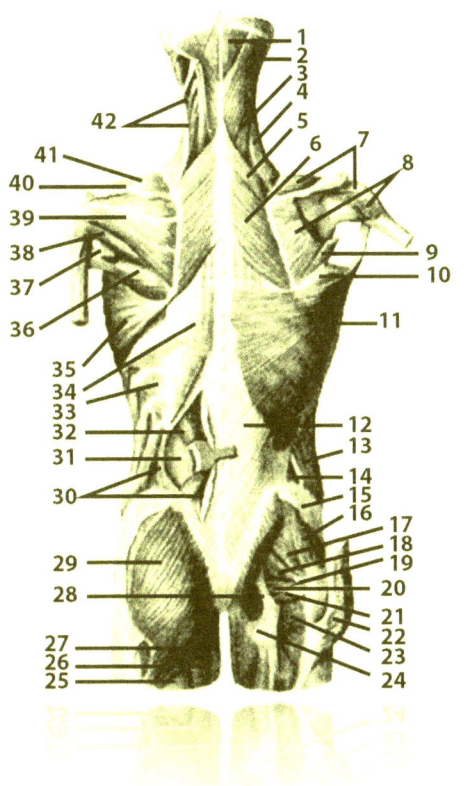

25 – biceps thigh muscle 598 617 329817
26 – semitendinous muscle 549 381 714 817
27 – greater adductor muscle 374 841 219 471
28 – sacrotuberal ligament 316 497 218 914
30 – surface leaf of fudo-lumbar fascia (the projection with the side flap) 494 848 514 216
31 – deep leaf of thoracolumbar fascia 481 319 614 714
32 – erector muscle of spine (drawn to the medial side) 598 748 519 491
33 – inferior posterior serratus muscle 549 317 919 817
34 – fudo-lumbar fascia 529 317 919 817
35 – anterior serratus muscle 219 475 819 355
36 – greater circular muscle 849 516 319 478
37 – long head of the triceps brachii muscle (part of image) 514 819 498 614
38 – minor circular muscle 498 518 491 748
39 – abdominal muscle 894 314 818 574
40 – spine of scapula 498 712 328 822
41 – supraspinatus muscle 312 214 812 514
42 – muscle lifting the shoulder-blade (drawn to the side) 214 317 914 717

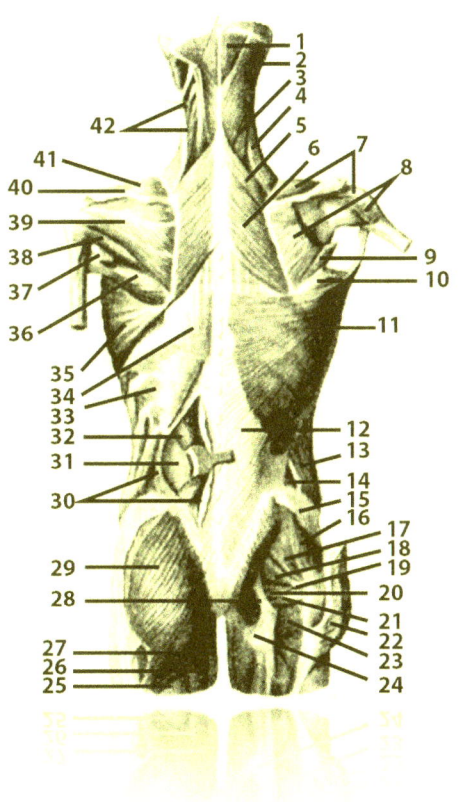

*Fig. 82 Muscles of the back and neck 498 549 618 714 (muscles and bones of the shoulder girdle are not shown):*

1 – semispinal muscle of head 914 217 218 498
2 – Belt muscle of head 298 742 279 488
3 – superior rear serratus muscle 898 549 694 714
4 – Belt muscle of neck 216 498 948 741
5 – external intercostal muscles 398 591 294 168
6 – iliocostal muscle of back 319 647 218 471
7 – longissimus muscle of back 497 549 819 714
8 – awned muscle 396 891 319 471
9 – inferior posterior serratus muscle 549 317 919 817
10 – latissimus dorsi muscle (part of the picture, turned aside 429 318 829 998
11 – aponeurosis of the latissimus dorsi 549 718 219 478
12 – lumbar triangle 894 568 514 811
13 – the iliac crest 894 547 218 471
14 – abdominal internal oblique muscle 398 217 818 417
15 – external oblique muscle of abdomen 529 312 419 272
16 – thoracolumbar fascia 584 317 019 641
17 – nuchal ligament 589 691 319 714

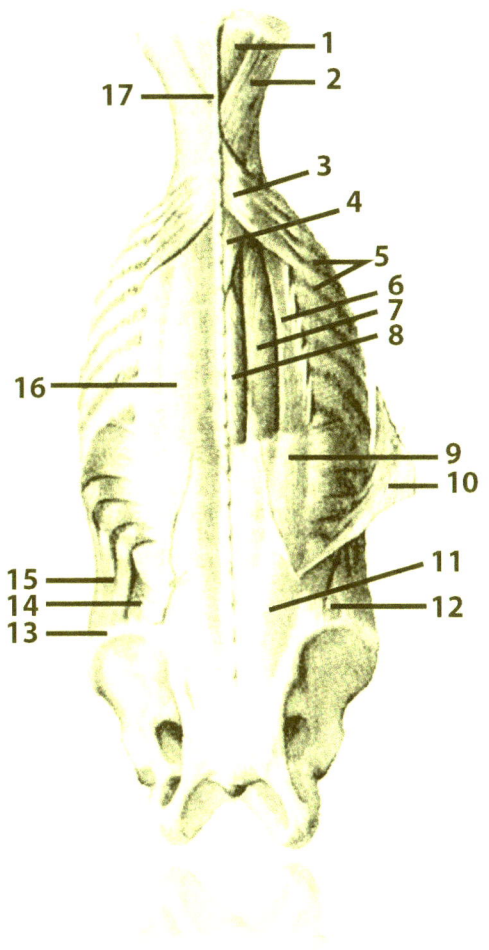

***Fig. 83 iliocostal muscle 314 841 619 714:***
1 – iliocostal muscle 314 841 619 714
2 – iliocostal muscle of neck 491 481 471 819
3 – iliocostal muscle of back 584 461 489 714
4 – iliocostal muscle of loin 578 714 218 417

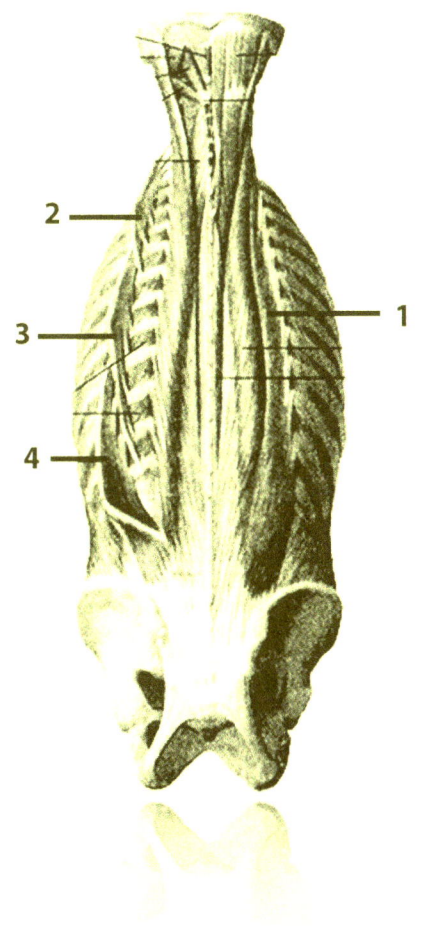

***Fig. 84 The deep muscles of the back and neck 498 714 219 614:***

1 – semispinal muscles of the head 914 217 218 498
2 – minor posterior rectus muscle of head 219 817 819 227
3 – superior oblique muscle of head 218 417 918 817
4 – larger posterior rectus muscle of head 594 318 614 715
5 – lower oblique muscle of head 218 317 918 227
6 – semispinal muscle of head (part of the picture, turned aside) 914 217 218 498
7 – semispinal neck muscle 319 714 218 412
8 – semispinal muscle of back 318 694 218 421
9 – the muscles that raise the ribs 689 714 298 514
10 – intertransverse muscles 519 314 819 312
11 – leaf of deep thoracolumbar fascia 481 319 614 714
12 – transverse abdominal muscle 555 813 915 513
13 – multifidus muscle 549 781 219 471
14 – wing of ilium 529 301 229 721
15 – iliocostal muscle 364 712 819 418
16 – longissimus muscle 589 641 289 714
17 – external intercostal muscles 369 581 298 471
18 – longissimus muscle of neck 699 186 019 491
19 – interspinous neck muscles 489 617 819 398
20 – longissimus muscle of head 389 497 368 141

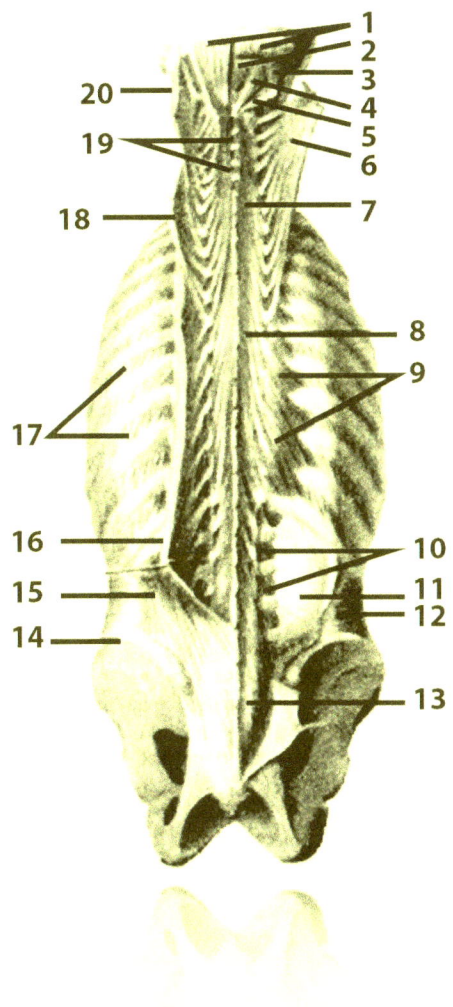

# FEMALE PELVIS 494 714 516 841
## Female sex organs 519 814 089 319

*Fig. 85 Female sex organs 519 814 089 319*
*(longitudinal median projection):*

1 – ovary 914 814 917 218
2 – Fallopian tube 619 718 316 214
3 – body of the uterus 689 514 218 471
4 – bladder 219 389 998 419
5 – hip bone (part of image) 214 317 918 227
6 – urethra 329 487 948 216
7 – clitoris 689 568 319 818
8 – labia majora 598 711 008 512
9 – labia minora 319 016 789 498
10 – uterine cervix 894 581 948 164
11 – Rectum 598 714 898 314
12 – sacrum 514 716 814 226
13 – vagina 889 491 619 819
14 – anus 589 317 418 917

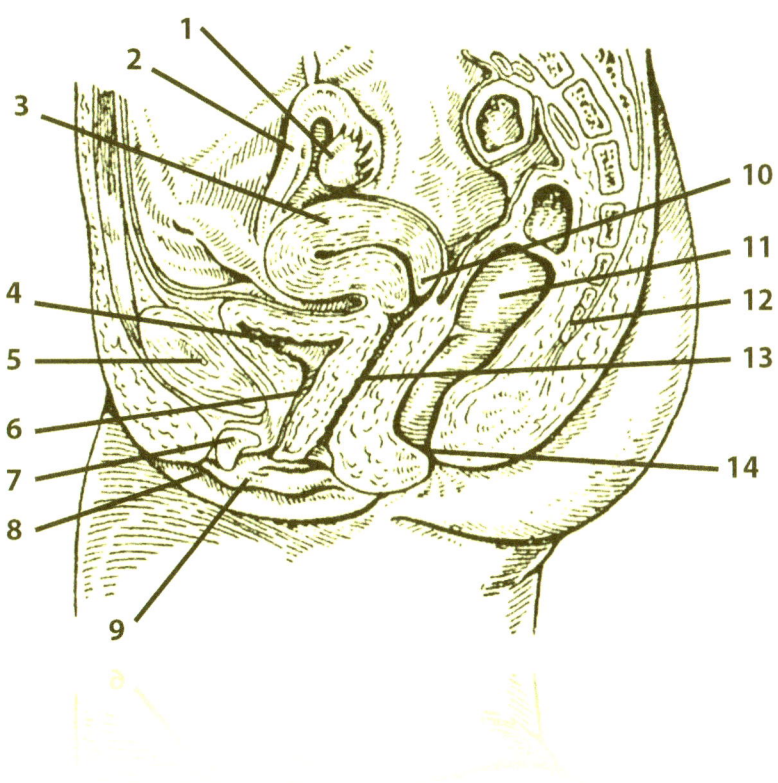

© Грабовой Г.П. 2002

**Female external genitalia 519 319 818 678**
**(Part 1, Fig. 124)**
**Internal female sex organs 419 219 808 319**

*Fig. 86 internal female sex organs 419 219 808 319:*

1 – vagina 889 491 619 819
2 – vaginal portion of the cervix 548 988 581 497
3 – cervical canal 614 891 719 489
4 – Isthmus 549 691 289 784
5 – uterine cavity 318 688 594 191
6 – uterine fundus 984 016 501 348
7 – wall of the uterus 841 369519 471
8 – Fallopian tube 619 718 316 214
9 – ovary 914 814 917 218
10 – interstitial portion of the tube 584 199 598 641
11 – isthmic part of the tube 589 612 319 471
12 – ampullar part of the tube 894 316 498 561
13 – fimbriae tubes 589 617 289 748
14 – sacro-uterine ligament 598 361 298 471
15 – ligament of the ovary 584 216 298 497
16 – funnel-pelvic ligament 294 147 284 641
17 – broad ligament 549 581 369 471
18 – round ligament 948 371 296 497
19 – projection of the ovary with follicles and corpus luteum 498 316 478 471
20 – parovarium 891 368 194 364

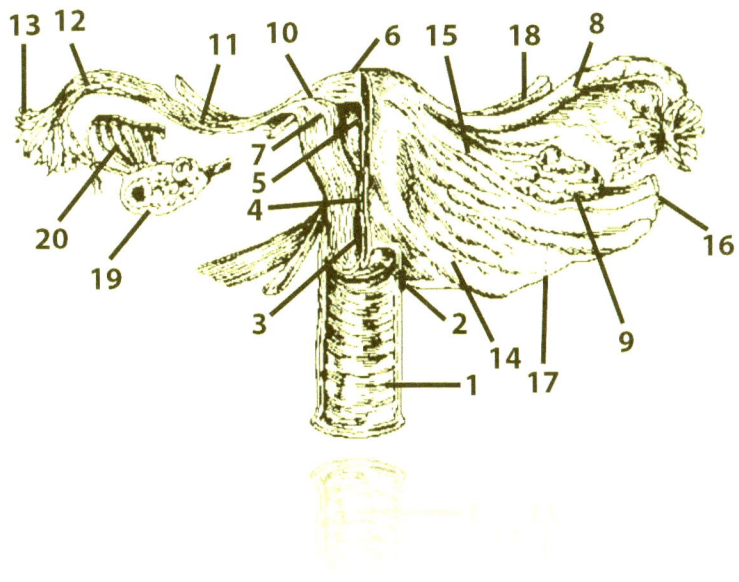

*Fig. 87 Schematic representation of the longitudinal projection of the ovary (a) and lateral projections of the uterus (b):*

a:

1 – primary follicles 498 518 818 491

2 – growing follicle 898 648 218 471

3 – white body 497 614 201 498

4 – Graaf bubble 481 684 371 016

5 – corpus luteum 818 401 616 214

b:

1 – uterine fundus 984 016 501 348

2 – uterine cavity 318 688 594 191

3 – body of the uterus 689 514 218 471

4 – uterine cervix 894 581 948 164

5 – the outer layer of the uterus, serous membrane (perimetrium) 848 147 218 417

6 – the middle layer of the uterus, the muscular layer (myometrium) 198 316 949 101

7 – the inner layer of the uterus, the mucous membrane (endometrium) 698 317 281 488

8 – Fallopian tube 619 718 316 214

9 – ovary 914 814 917 218

10 – vagina 889 491 619 819

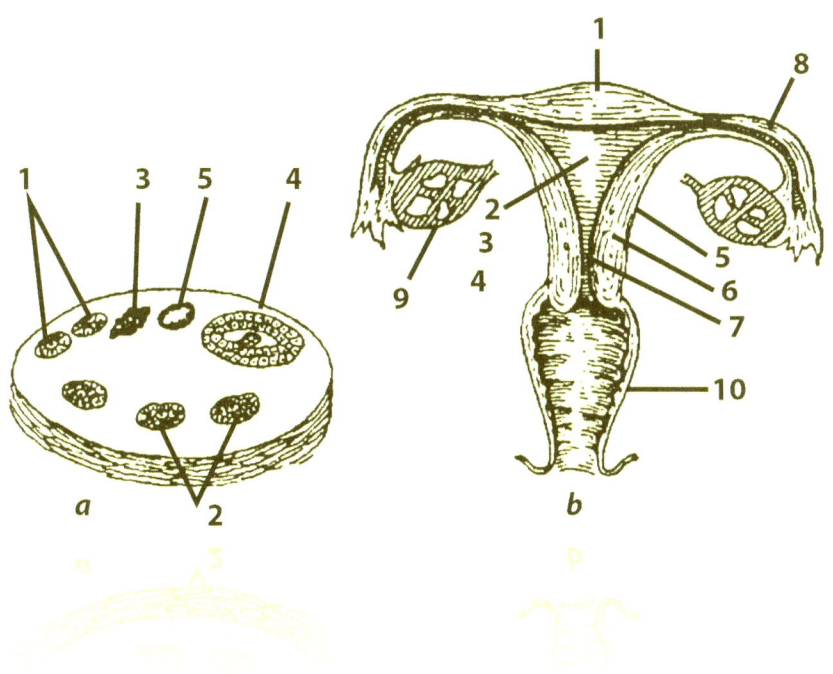

© Грабовой Г.П. 2002

**MAMMARY GLAND 648317219491**

*Fig. 88 Structure and holography of mammary gland:*

1 – lateral axillary lymph node 497 218 217 498

2 – the axillary artery 694 718 217 491

3 – axillary vein 849 716 218 471

4 – brachial plexus 312 314 512 214

5 – central axillary lymph node 648 516 201 505

6 – apical axillary lymph nodes 618 471 298 741

7 – supraclavicular lymph nodes 598 641 264 271

8a – lateral thoracic artery 598 722 918 213

8b – lateral thoracic vein 584 317 248 517

9 – sternal lymph nodes 649 318 714 618

10 – plexus of blood and lymphatic vessels 510 314 784 617

11 – a branch of the internal thoracic artery to the mammary gland 479 841 589 641

12 – areola 394 647 198 518

13 – milk ducts 471 691 284 714

14 – lateral arterial branches of mammary gland 691 014 398 517

15 – pectoral axillary lymph nodes 749 148 519 618

16 – subscapular lymph nodes 184 816 014 214

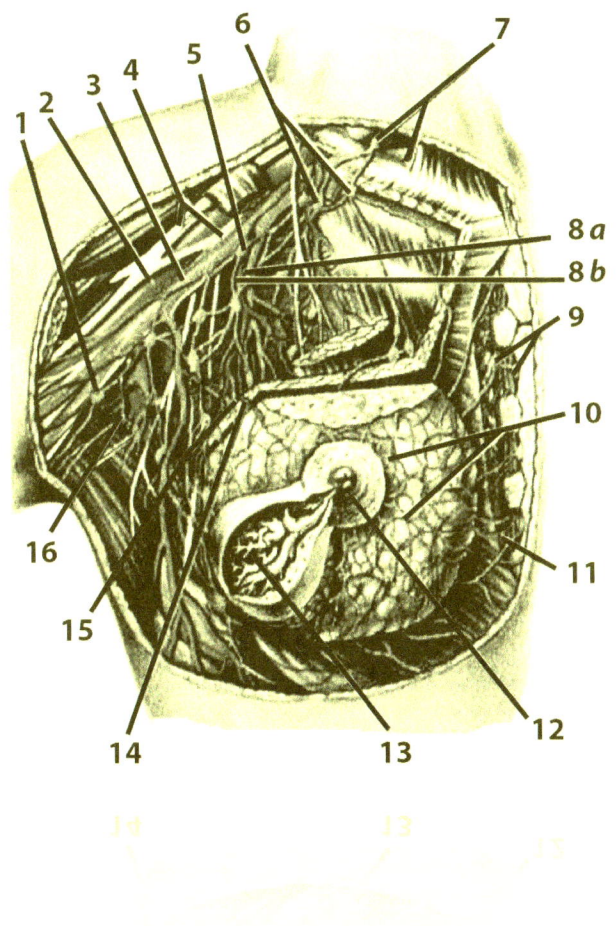

***Fig. 89 Anatomy of mammary gland:***
1 – muscle cells 494 816 319 481
2 – cells secreting milk 859 169 794 217
3 – milk ducts 471 691 284 714
4 – lactiferous sinuses 584 316 219 478
5 – nipple 894 181 319 718
6 – areola 394 647 198 518
7 – Montgomery glands 491 819 488 514
8 – alveoli 614 819 319 714
9 – supporting and adipose tissue 898 617 219 419

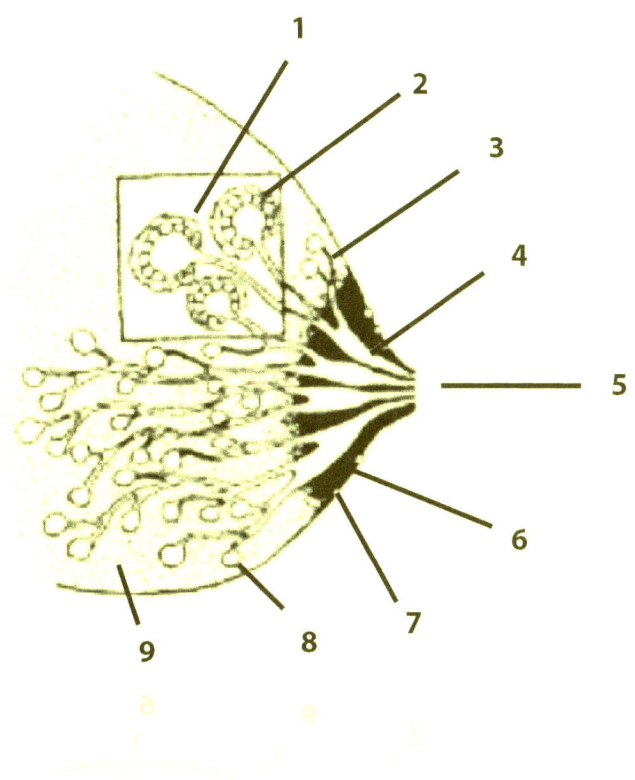

# The cardiovascular system (continued) 214 700 819 891

## Fig. 90 Head and neck arteries
## (right side) (continued) 518 422 819 312:

1 – subclavian artery (right) 598 317 819 227
2 – costocervical trunk 549 641 898 714
3 – the highest intercostal artery 589 716 549 818
4 – Thyrocervical trunk 519 317 919 288
5 – suprascapular artery 529 317 419 817
6 – deep cervical artery 598 714 898 716
7 – ascending cervical artery 749 814 719 414
8 – VI - cervical vertebra 568 314 819 714
9 – pharyngeal branches 498 217 228 417
10 – common carotid artery (right) 919 421 818 728
11 – vertebral artery (cervical part) 498 714 319 716
12 – spinal branches 584 314 819 417
13 – internal carotid artery 549 712 810 248
14 – ascending pharyngeal artery 496 598 317 641
15 – occipital artery 581 214 608 491
16 – vertebral artery (cervico-occipital part) 918 317 948 561
17 – vertebral artery (right) (intracranial portion) 364 819 498 471
18 – vertebral artery (left) (intracranial portion) 364 819 498 471
19 – inferior tympanic artery 894 168 941 987
20 – posterior meningeal artery 594 162 398 714

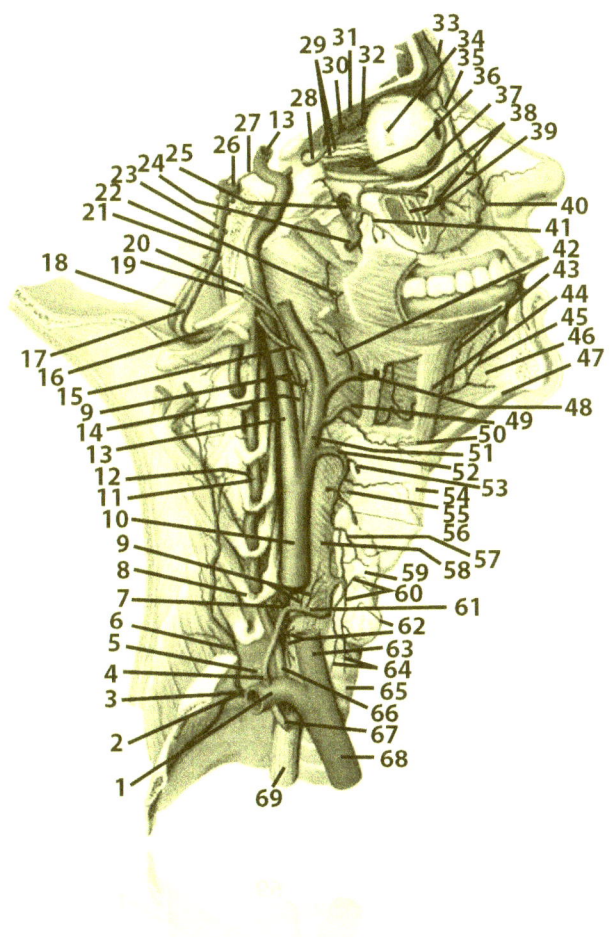

© Грабовой Г.П. 2002 215

21 – clivus of the skull base 319 778 219 228
22 – tonsillar branch 895 316 498 471
23 – basilar artery 851 478 594 814
24 – maxillary artery 648 517 284 917
25 – wedge palatine artery 598 491 374 816
26 – posterior cerebral artery 594 361 809 491
27 – posterior communicating artery 548 641 298 781
28 – ophthalmic artery 649 718 549 641
29 – posterior short ciliary arteries 496 391 898 671
30 – posterior ethmoid artery 594 716 298 491
31 – supraorbital artery 594 617 548 518
32 – anterior ethmoid artery 698 713 294 168
33 – supratrochlear artery 798 791 694 814
34 – lateral rectus muscle of eye 328 421 898 712
35 – dorsal nasal artery 368 142 598 714
36 – Long posterior ciliary arteries 581 641 294 818
37 – inferior oblique muscle of eye 319 618 204 881
38 – infraorbital artery 898 048 319 061
39 – anterior superior cellular arteries 364 181 298 471
40 – angular artery 288 919 069 789
41 – posterior superior cellular artery 549 161 298 191
42 – ascending palatine artery 581 494 549 618
43 – deep artery of tongue 319 694 384 716
44 – hyo-lingual muscle 368 142 498 641
45 – sublingual artery 784 981 294 671
46 – genioglossal muscle 218 614 319 718

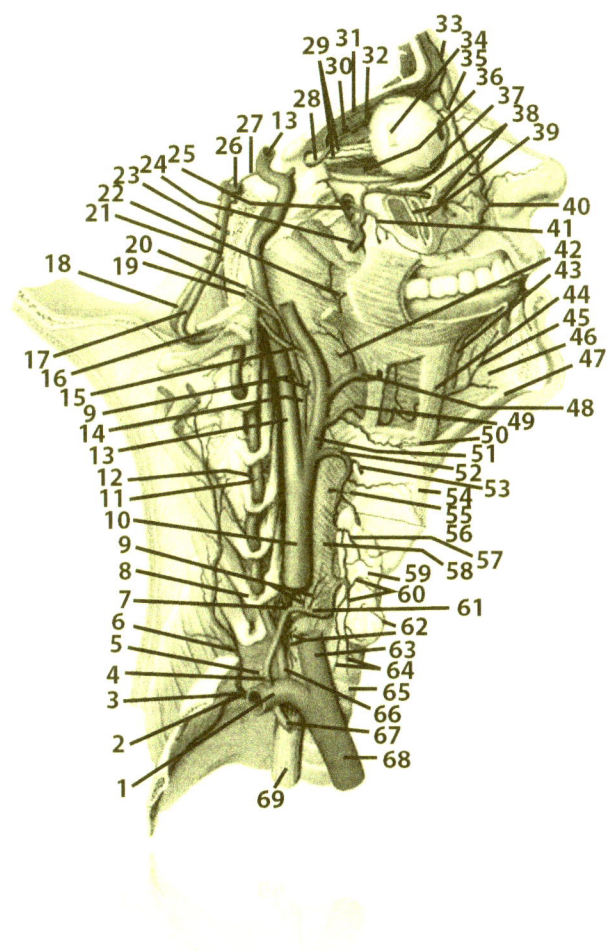

47 – geniohyoid muscle 498 694 819 671

48 – facial artery 219 061 234 890

49 – lingual artery 498 519 401 209

50 – suprahyoid branch 691 318 464 148

51– external carotid artery 510 469 148 712

52 – superior thyroid artery 519 513 719 313

53 – superior laryngeal artery 389 461 894 171

54 – thyrohyoid membrane 584 691 219 478

55 – sternocleidomastoid branch 519 614 431 548

56 – anterior branch of superior thyroid artery 698 517 401 469

57 – dorsal branch of the superior thyroid arteries 014 981 564 168

58 – gulp 519 987 319 427

59 – thyroid gland 829 319 409 819

60 – glandular branches 149 816 013 009

61 – inferior thyroid artery 518 377 918 478

62 – oesophageal branches 519 512 319 812

63 – common carotid artery 894 317 212 847

64 – tracheal branches 919 810 499 310

65 – Trachea 429 318 919 888

66 – vertebral artery (prevertebral part) 109 467 219 891

67 – internal thoracic artery 598 341 818 941

68 – brachiocephalic trunk 998 301 248 227

69 – Esophagus 598 381 698 711

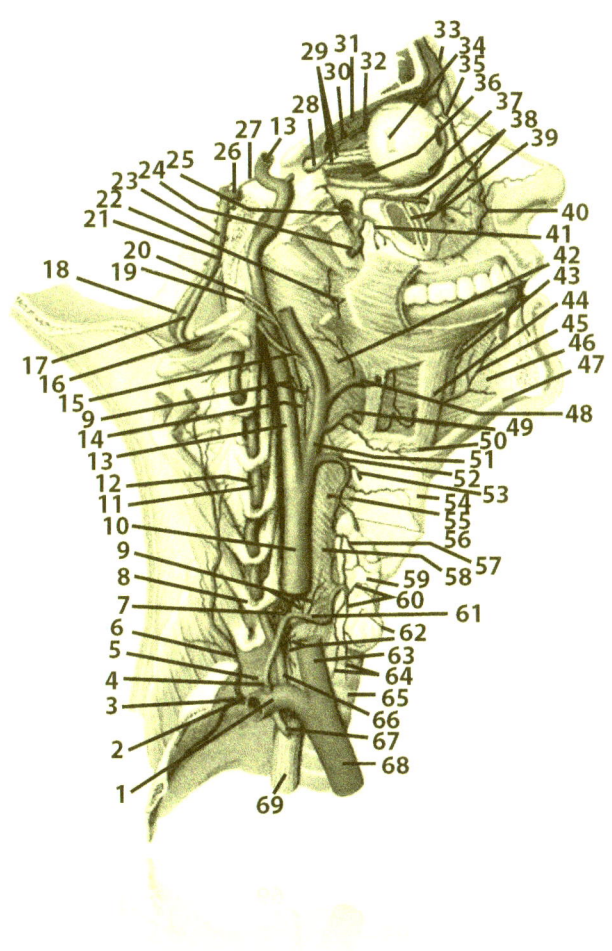

219

***Fig. 91 The veins of the head and neck (right side) 598 716 319 816:***
1 – transverse vein of neck 814 416 214 319
2 – spinal vein of 146 472 019 541
3 – anterior vertebral vein of 109 516 918 416
4 – accessory vertebral vein of 210 341 907 654
5 – external jugular vein 594 716 814 516
6 – vein of deep neck 801 498 548 617
7 – facial vein of 599 715 819 316
8 – external vertebral venous plexus 421 054 329 891
9 – postmaxillary vein of 364 817 384 199
10 – superior jugular bulb 448 546 891 479
11 – occipital vein 914 712 298 267
12 – condylar emissary vein 648 513 694 817
13 – posterior auricular vein 368 198 549 617
14 – mastoid emissary vein 391 849 501 011
15 – sigmoid sinus 109 516 397 894
16 – occipital sinus 012 126 094 791
17 – the transverse sinus 549 716 398 471
18 – occipital emissary vein 548 617 294 581
19 – torcular Herophili 364 814 501 122
20 – inferior petrosal sinus 284 368 149 017
21 – superior petrosal sinus 019 596 394 717
22 – straight sinus 849 712 646 181
23 – superficial temporal veins 694 513 814 216
24 – inferior sagittal sinus 814 316 219 497
25 – greater vein of brain 498 142 549 617

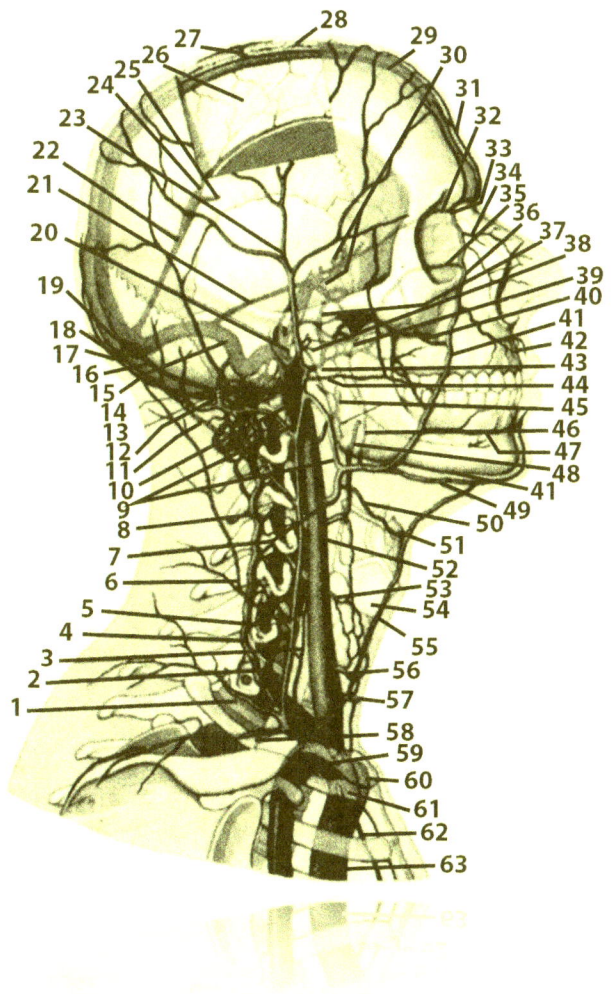

26 – falx of cerebrum 001 918 021 378
27 – parietal emissary vein 349 161 894 717
28 – diploic veins 148 564 219 617
29 – superior sagittal sinus 914 715 514 292
30 – cavernous sinus 846 139 948 581
31 – vein supratrochlear 819 621 398 471
32 – superior ophthalmic vein 909 610 549 798
33 – nasofrontal vein 514 369 129 710
34 – external nasal vein 319 481 589 671
35 – inferior ophthalmic vein 149 678 148 591
36 – Corner vein 693 146 590 310
37 – middle meningeal vein 018 531 219 641
38 – parotid gland veins 516 949 140 510
39 – pterygoid plexus 591 248 791 260
40 – deep facial vein 309 864 194 971
41 – facial vein 599 715 819 316
42 – superior labial vein 504 361 309 584
43 – maxillary vein 598 314 818 914
44 – transverse face vein 698 713 294 167
45 – pharyngeal veins 019 818 594 614
46 – palatine vein 548 316 819 471
47 – lower lip vein 547 218 599 641
48 – lingual vein 318 586 389 471
49 – submental vein 194 368 594 817
50 – superior thyroid vein 648 471 201 199
51 – hyoid bone 549 316 219 841

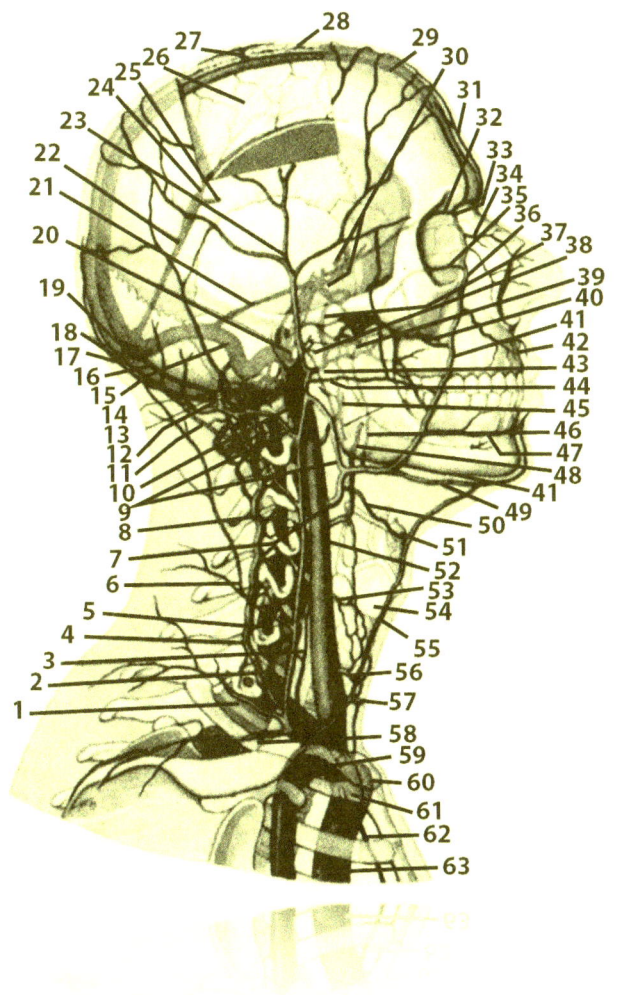

52 – internal jugular vein 598 612 719 322

53 – middle thyroid vein 814 017 201 849

54 – thyroid cartilage 588 421 388 711

55 – anterior jugular vein 368 541 291 479

56 – inferior thyroid vein 108 641 294 719

57 – inferior bulb of jugular vein 512 621 221 848

58 – suprascapular vein 548 571 818 548

59 – subclavian vein 598 317 898 214

60 – brachiocephalic vein (left) 219 378 919 278

61 – brachiocephalic vein (right) 219 378 919 278

62 – internal thoracic vein 491 316 894 198

63 – superior hollow vein 398 712 988 012

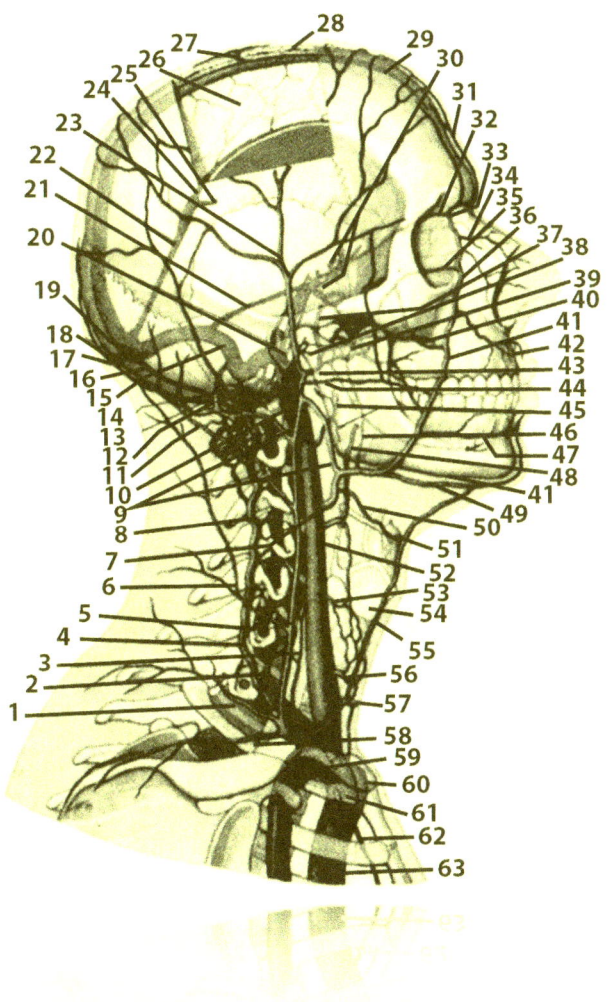

© Грабовой Г.П. 2002

*Fig. 92 The arteries of the brain (bottom view) 498 641 898 478:*

1 – branch of the cerebellar tonsils 549 641 891 748

2 – posterior inferior cerebellar artery 469 718 549 641

3 – hypoglossal nerve 548 321 555 678

4 – cranial nerve 584 647 289 741

5 – anterior inferior cerebellar artery 598 691 798 641

6 – nodulus 897 567 971 319

7 – choroid plexus of the fourth ventricle 694 167 298 547

8 – artery of bridge 467 589 196 318

9 – superior cerebellar artery 361 948 594 161

10 – oculomotor nerve 519217519217

11 – optic tract 519 218 919 245

12 – hypothalamus funnel 519 211 919 000

13 – optic chiasm 010 216 319517

14 – olfactory triangle 518 642 319 716

15 – olfactory tract 718 217 458 917

16 – olfactory bulb 024 312 598 742

17 – anterior cerebral arteries (postcommunicational part) 468 514 398 617

18 – medial orbital-frontal branch 518 641 201 009

19 – anterior communicating artery 641 478 594 641

20 – anterior cerebral arteries (precommunicational part) 584 061 412 011

21 – lateral fronto-basal artery 618 531 214 712

22 – internal carotid artery 549 712 810 248

23 – insular arteries 518 714 316 214

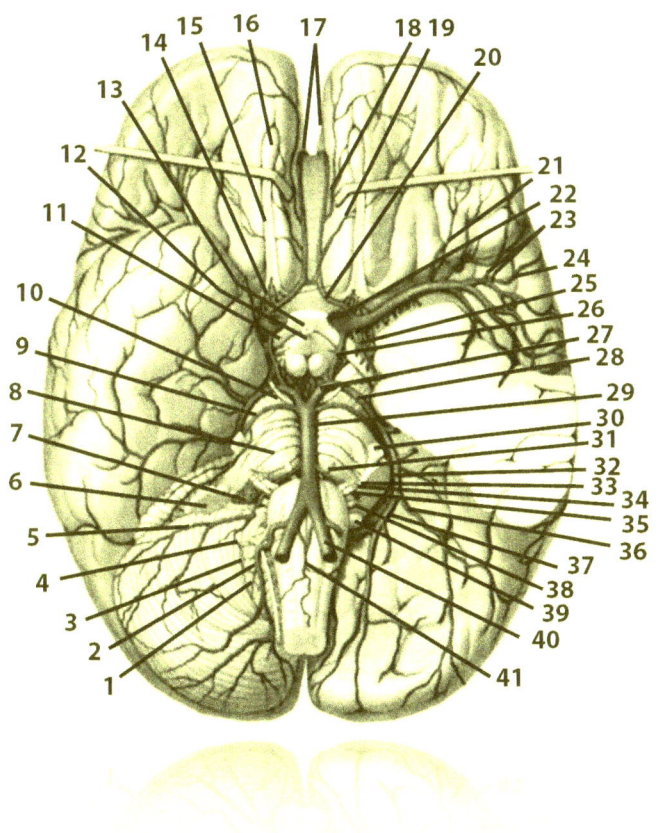

© Грабовой Г.П. 2002

227

24 – middle cerebral artery 496 491 817 514
25 – anterior villous artery of vascular plexus 491 316 498 714
26 – posterior communicating artery 548 641 298 781
27 – posterior cerebral artery (precommunicational part) 548 641 798 521
28 – posterior cerebral artery (postcommunicational part) 316 594 218 749
29 – basilar artery 851 478 594 814
30 – trigeminal nerve 549 319 818 711
31 – abducent nerve 514 517 214 812
32 – posterior cerebral artery (temporal part) 498 671 291 491
33 – intermediate nerve 219 381 648 719
34 – facial nerve 999 811 319 211
35 – vestibulocochlear nerve 548 217 918 421
36 – lateral occipital artery (final part) 619 012 504 794
37 – medial occipital artery (final part) 581 704 916 219
38 – glossopharyngeal nerve 519 371 214 572
39 – vagus nerve 489 981 728 221
40 – vertebral artery (left) (intracranial portion) 364 819 498 471
41 – anterior spinal artery 617 281 707 914

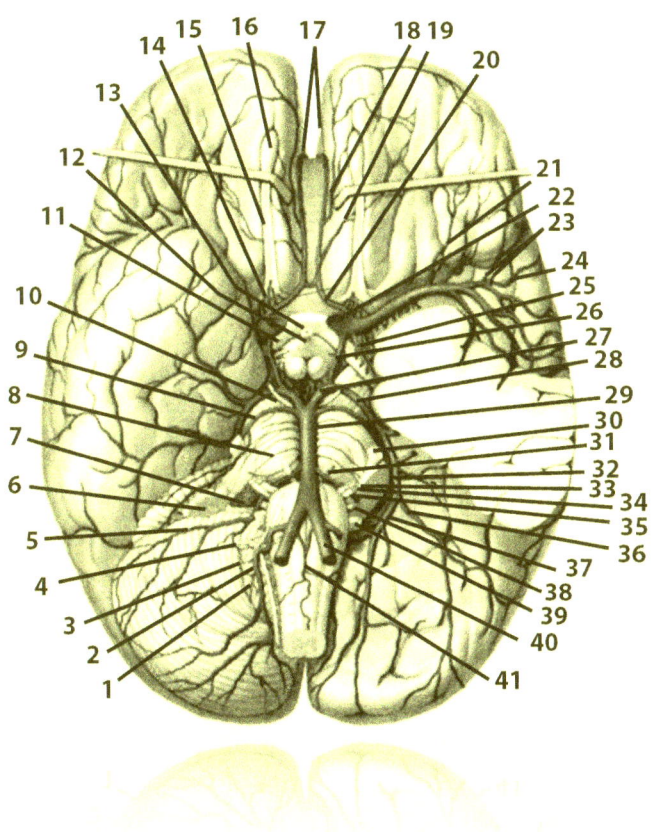

## Fig. 93 The arteries of the brain (medial surface) 469 518 716 491:

1 – intermediate-medial frontal branch 498 617 319 478
2 – anterior cerebral artery 317 498 689 171
3 – posteromedial frontal branch (anterior cerebral artery) 781 496 319 641
4 – groove belt 579 312 919 021
5 – groove of the corpus callosum 248 312 848 212
6 – Belt branch (anterior cerebral artery) 497 101 398 712
7 – corpus callosum 498 712 328 071
8 – fornix 648 314 589 716
9 – paracentral branch (anterior cerebral artery) 364 817 294 317
10 – precuneus branch (anterior cerebral artery) 694 171 894 214
11 – parietal-occipital sulcus 691 378 549 617
12 – parietal-occipital branch (posterior cerebral artery) 691 314 291 491
13 – parietal branch (posterior cerebral artery) 814 216 497 218
14 – occipital-temporal branch (posterior cerebral artery) 514 618 319 481
15 – calcarine branch (posterior cerebral artery) 564 814 219 417
16 – calcarine sulcus 214 318 414 888
17 – posterior cerebral artery 594 361 809 491
18 – medial occipital artery 581 704 916 219
19 – posterior temporal branches (posterior cerebral artery) 649 371 298 481
20 – pineal gland (epiphysis) 489 641 399 042
21 – quadrigeminal plate (quadrigeminal bodies) 514 317 818 212

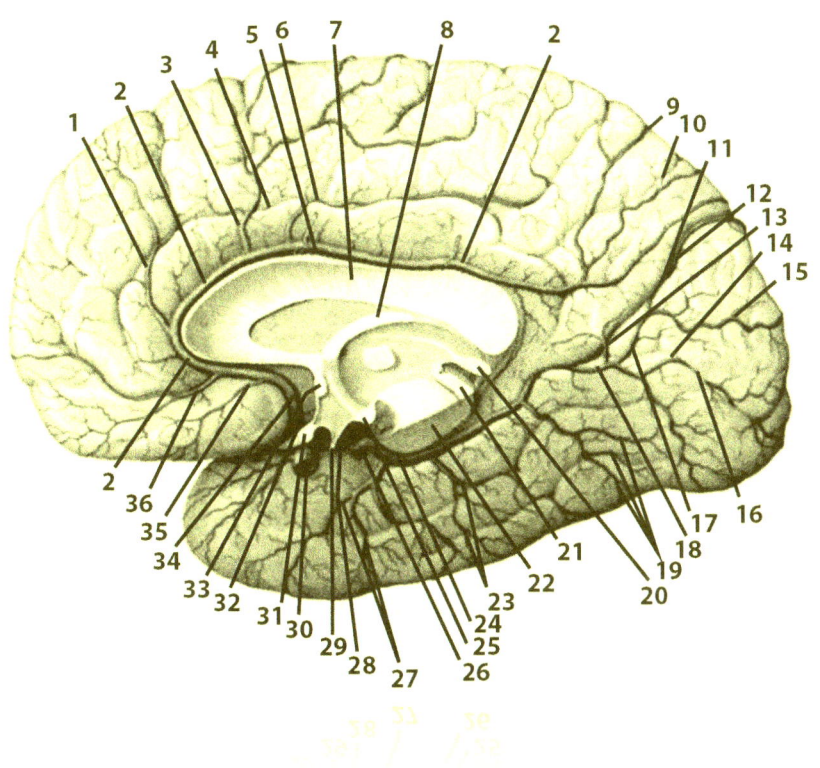

22 – cerebral peduncle 918 412 818 212

23 – intermediate temporal branches 549 648 391 361

24 – lateral occipital artery 496 819 716 478

25 – mammillary body 534 817 214 712

26 – posterior cerebral artery (temporal part) 498 671 291 491

27 – anterior temporal branches (lateral occipital artery) 648 531 219 471

28 – posterior communicating artery 548 641 298 781

29 – groove on the bottom of the funnel III of cerebral ventricle 568 016 219 014

30 – internal carotid artery 549 712 810 248

31 – optic chiasm 010 216 319 517

32 – terminal plate 048 541 298 647

33 – anterior commissure 389 691 974 846

34 – anterior communicating artery 641 478 594 641

35 – medial frontal-basal artery (medial orbital-frontal branch) 518 641 201 009

36 – anteromedial frontal branch (anterior cerebral artery) 698 142 489 716

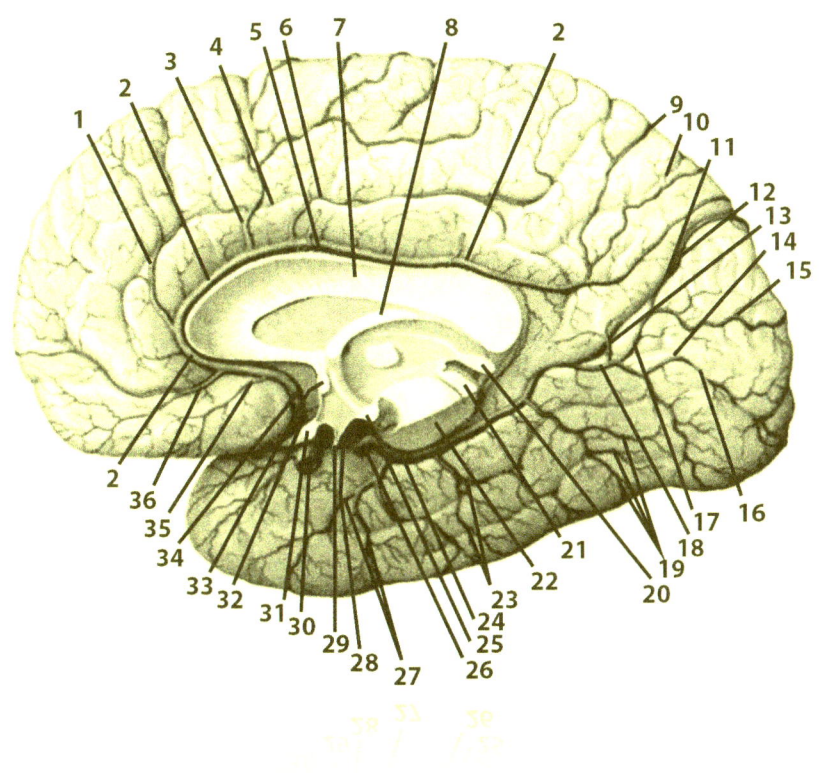

***Fig. 94 The arteries of the brain***
***(upper lateral surface) 469 471 898 417:***

1 – posterior inferior cerebellar artery 469 718 549 641
2 – Cerebellum 828 219 328 299
3 – occipital lobe 519 617 298 714
4 – angular gyrus artery 519 617 289 741
5 – posterior parietal artery 164 816 319 471
6 – anterior parietal artery 014 146 214 814
7 – parietal lobe 618 041 894 141
8 – artery of postcentral sulcus 102 348 410 514
9 – artery of central sulcus 648 318 489 316
10 – artery of precentral sulcus 584 216 218 714
11 – frontal lobe 316 618 319 417
12 – lateral fronto-basal artery 618 531 214 712
13 – island 584 216 298 741
14 – insular arteries 518 714 316 214
15 – middle cerebral artery 496 491 817 514
16 – anterior temporal artery 689 371 298 681
17 – middle temporal artery 618 591 294 317
18 – temporal lobe 564 931 298 714
19 – posterior temporal artery 548 721 296 397
20 – basilar artery 851 478 594 814
21 – Bridge 248 317 284 271
22 – vertebral artery (right) (intracranial portion) 364 819 498 471

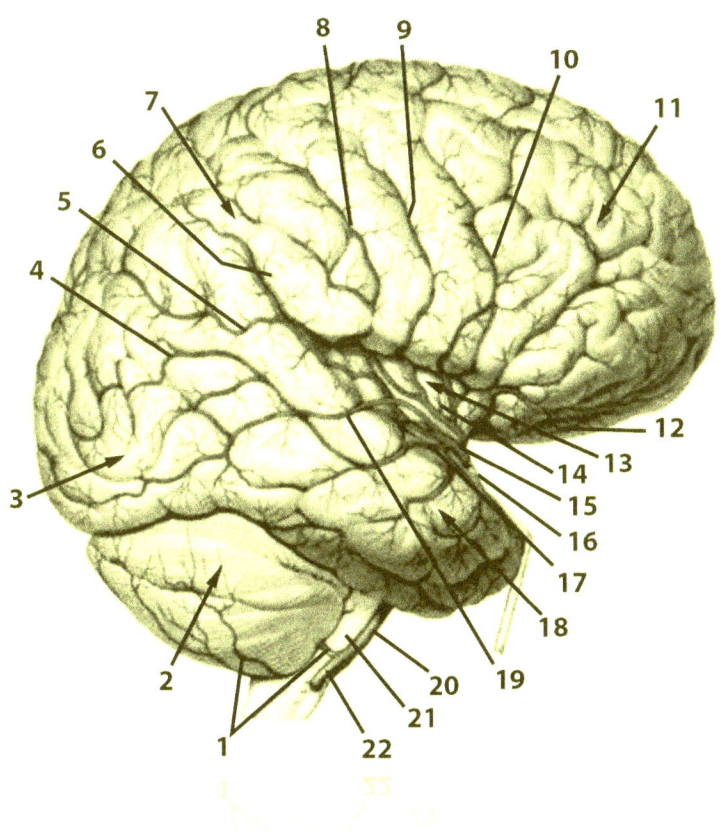

*Fig. 95 Superficial cerebral veins*
*(upper lateral surface) 649 712 519 747:*

1 – sigmoid sinus 109 516 397 894
2 – upper petrosal sinus 019 596 394 717
3 – posterior auricular vein 368 198 549 617
4 – transverse sinus 549 716 398 471
5 – occipital vein 914 712 298 267
6 – mastoid emissary vein 391 849 501 011
7 – occipital emissary vein 548 617 294 581
8 – occipital veins 789 621 298 491
9 – dura mater of the brain 333 489 312 289
10 – parietal lobe 618 041 894 141
11 – lateral venous lacuna 569 317 398 471
12 – parietal vein 394 569 398 741
13 – superior sagittal sinus 914 715 514 292
14 – superior anastomotic vein 341 318 519 641
15 – frontal veins 361 384 219 471
16 – frontal lobe 316 618 319 417
17 – prefrontal veins 598 641 298 791
18 – superficial middle cerebral vein 694 178 394 516
19 – temporal lobe 564 931 298 714
20 – inferior anastomotic vein 391 568 914 918
21 – inferior cerebral veins 719 628 514 318
22 – inferior petrous sinus 284 368 149 017
23 – internal jugular vein 598 612 719 322

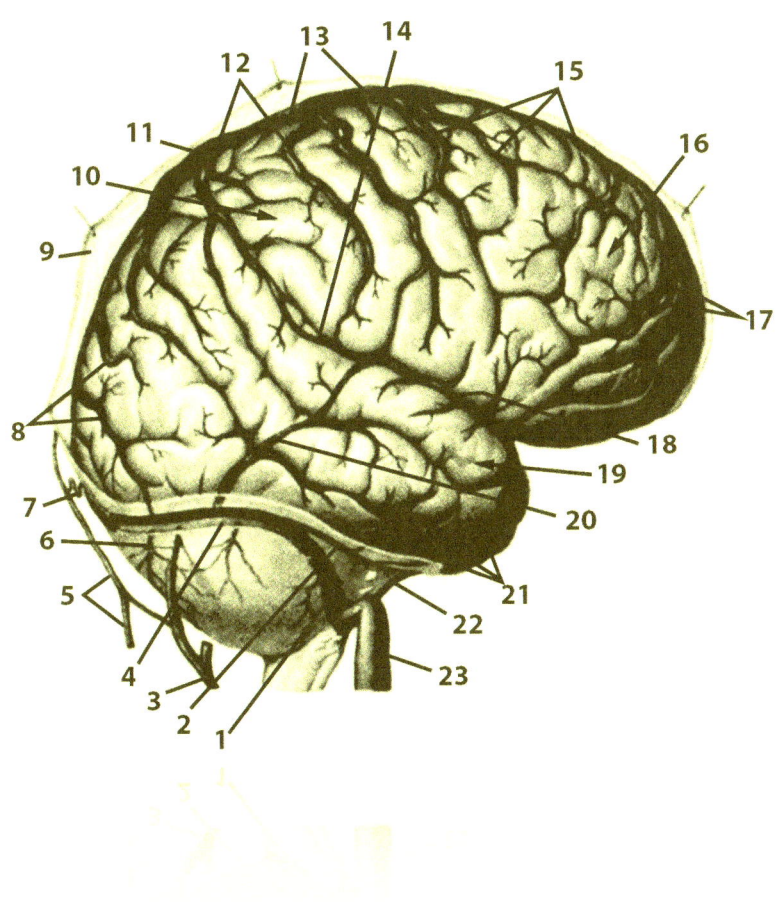

© Грабовой Г.П. 2002

*Fig. 96 sinuses of the dura mater 691 958 549 164:*
1 – basal vein 202 464 891 319
2 – large cerebral vein 498 142 549 617
3 – transverse sinus 549 716 398 471
4 – occipital sinus 012 126 094 791
5 – diploic veins 148 564 219 617
6 – sinus passages 364 814 501 122
7 – fourth ventricle 514 321 414 218
8 – straight sinus 849 712 646 181
9 – upper cerebral veins 519 316 489 718
10 – greater falciform process of the dura mater 364 815 398 574
11 – Bridge 248 317 284 271
12 – inner brain vein 541 219 319 471
13 – Vascular basis of III ventricle 584 217 284 917
14 – superior sagittal sinus 914 715 514 292
15 – lateral gaps 398 741 298 474
16 – superior villous vein 518 361 987 241
17 – inferior sagittal sinus 814 316 219 497
18 – superficial temporal vein 548 327 918 227
19 – parietal emissary vein 349 161 894 717
20 – superior thalamostriate veins 598 164 398 711
21 – lateral ventricle 649 140 508 914
22 – lamina of septum pellucidum 319 798 549 164
23 – knee of the corpus callosum 148 512 319 417
24 – anterior vein of septum pellucidum 849 617 219 514

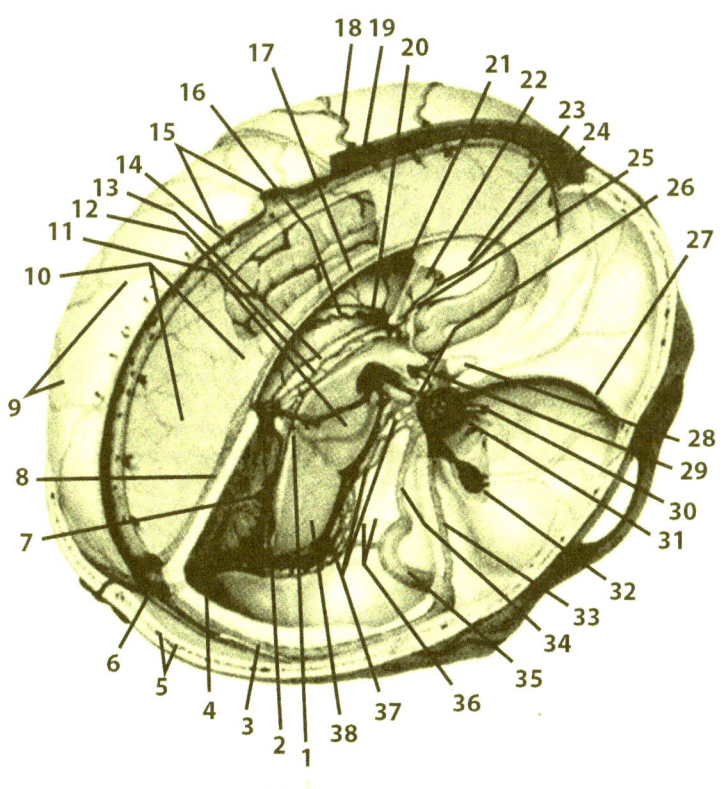

25 – column of fornix 168 794 598 716
26 – Intercavernous sinuses 514 019 598 411
27 – sphenoparietal sinus 514 312 619 718
28 – optic nerve 448 817 918 217
29 – internal carotid artery 549 712 810 248
30 – superficial middle cerebral vein 694 178 394 516
31 – cavernous sinus 846 139 948 581
32 – venous plexus of the foramen ovale 498 716 374 917
33 – superior petrosal sinus 019 596 394 717
34 – inferior petrous sinus 284 368 149 017
35 – sigmoid sinus 109 516 397 894
36 – venous plexus of hypoglossal canal 598 611 998 164
37 – basilar plexus 691 319 819 471
38 – medulla oblongata 514 417 814 217

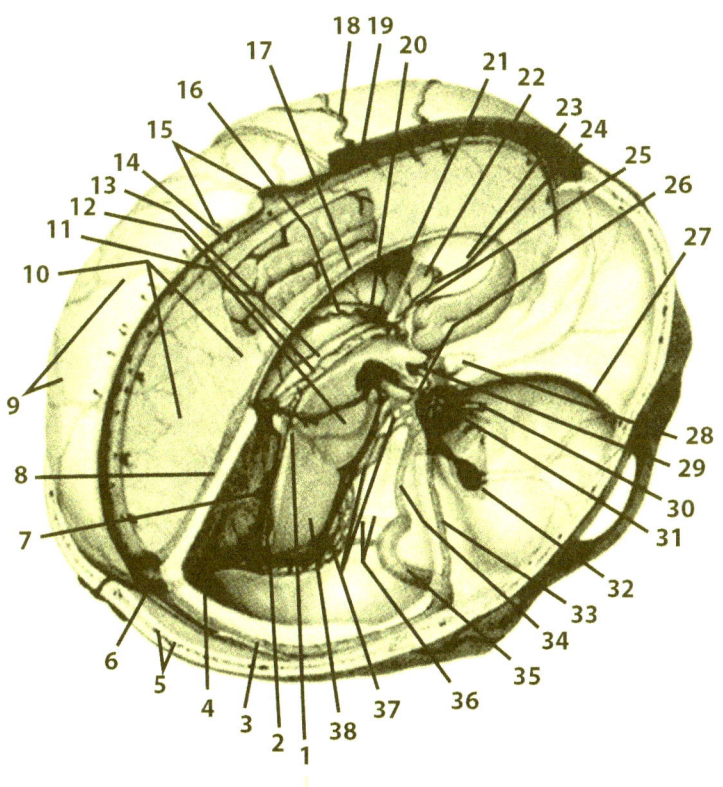

© Грабовой Г.П. 2002

241

## Arteries and veins of the heart 514 814 219 417

### Fig. 97 Arteries and veins of the heart (sternocostal surface) 514 814 219 417:

1 – right ventricle of the heart 598 371 988 011
2 – arterial cone 548 647 219 741
3 – right marginal branch of right coronary artery 518 617 219 419
4 – anterior cardiac veins 648 715 594 317
5 – intermediate atrial branches 594 781 978 471
6 – coronal sulcus 519 312 814 829
7 – branch of arterial cone 394 168 574 971
8 – right coronary artery 691 368 519 479
9 – right auricle of heart 598 714 321 898
10 – superior hollow vein 398 712 988 012
11 – ascending aorta 598 712 898 612
12 – right pulmonary artery 694 897 594 716
13 – brachiocephalic trunk 998 301 248 227
14 – common carotid artery (left) 428 712 488 913
15 – subclavian artery (left) 429 387 219 377
16 – aortic arch 219 877 549 277
17 – arterial ligament 519 481 319 818
18 – left pulmonary artery 691 318 497 541
19 – pulmonary trunk 519 421 819 221
20 – left auricle of heart 519 318 219 481
21 – left coronary artery 194 641 291 891
22 – circumflex branch of the left coronary artery 619 471 218 514

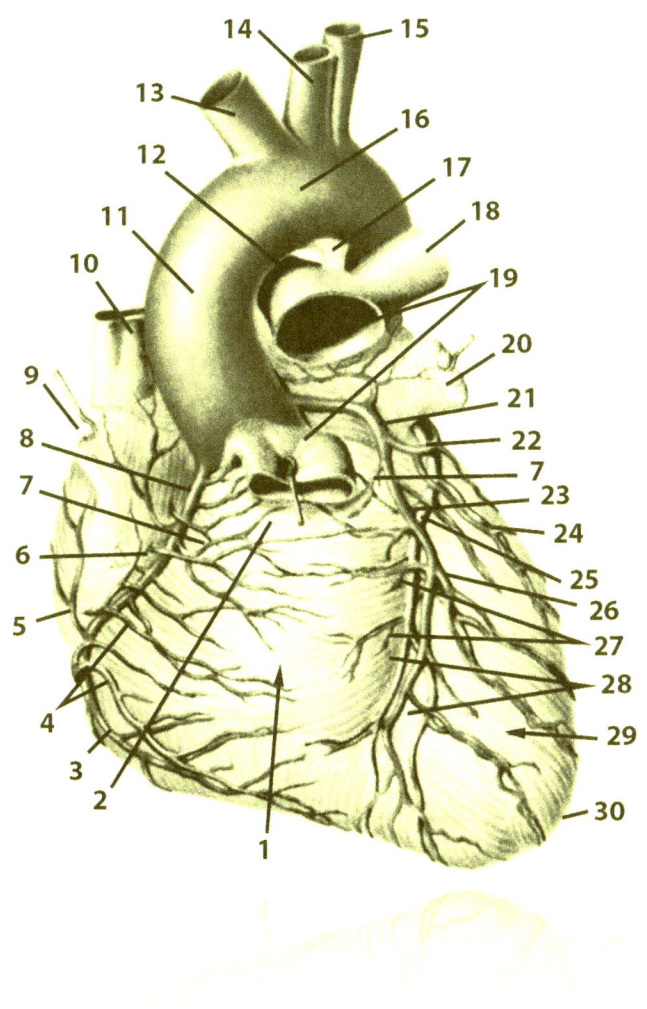

23 – anterior descending branch of the left coronary artery 364 891 291 471
24 – left marginal branch 589 714 210 481
25 – great cardiac vein 641 217 498 718
26 – lateral branch 491 316 218 714
27 – interventricular septal branches 691 314 219 718
28 – anterior descending furrow 909 817 398 787
29 – left ventricle 589 348 914 918
30 – apex of heart 519 421 899 321

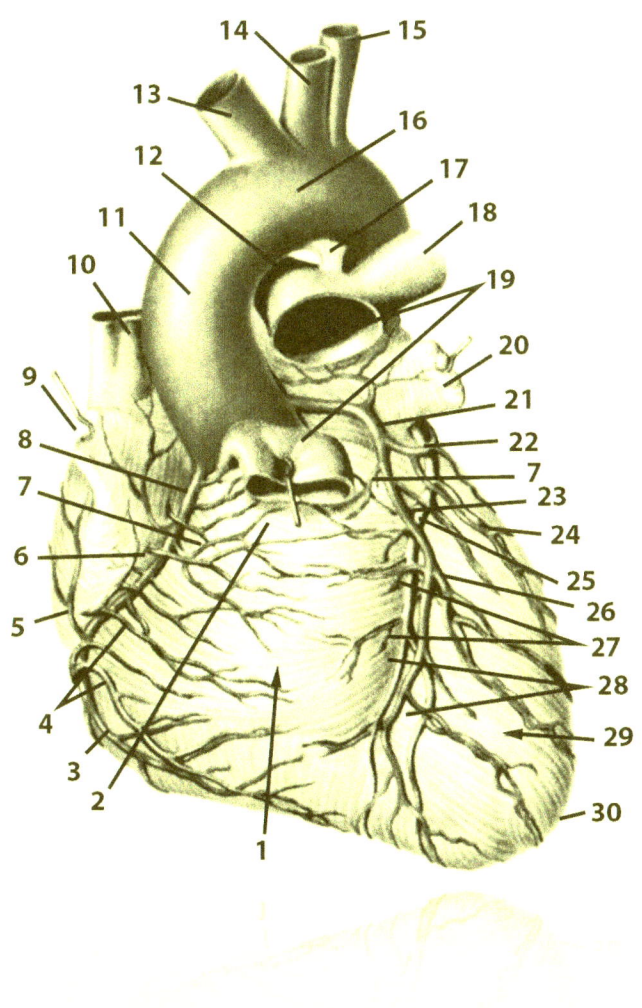

245

*Fig. 98 The arteries and veins of the heart (diaphragmatic surface) 514 816 914 317:*

1 – apex cardiac 519 421 899 321
2 – left ventricle 589 348 914 918
3 – anastomotic atrial branch 614 917 918 517
4 – left marginal branch 589 714 210 481
5 – posterior vein of left ventricular 429 318 719 888
6 – posterior branch of the left ventricle 467 548 219 741
7 – circumflex branch of the left coronary artery 619 471 218 514
8 – great cardiac vein 641 217 498 718
9 – oblique vein of the left atrium 598 714 319 814
10 – intermediate atrial branches 594 781 978 471
11a – left superior pulmonary vein 549 671 298 471
11b – left inferior pulmonary vein 598 649 219 714
12 – left atrium 518 712 314 887
13 – left pulmonary artery 697 108 889 491
14 – arterial ligament 519 481 319 818
15 – subclavian artery (left) 429 387 219 377
16 – common carotid artery (left) 428 712 488 913
17 – brachiocephalic trunk 998 301 248 227
18 – aortic arch 219 877 549 277
19 – superior hollow vein 398 712 988 012
20 – right pulmonary artery 694 897 594 716
21a – right superior pulmonary vein 691 894 319 712
21b – right inferior pulmonary vein 697 213 519 491
22 – right atrium 491 016 519 497

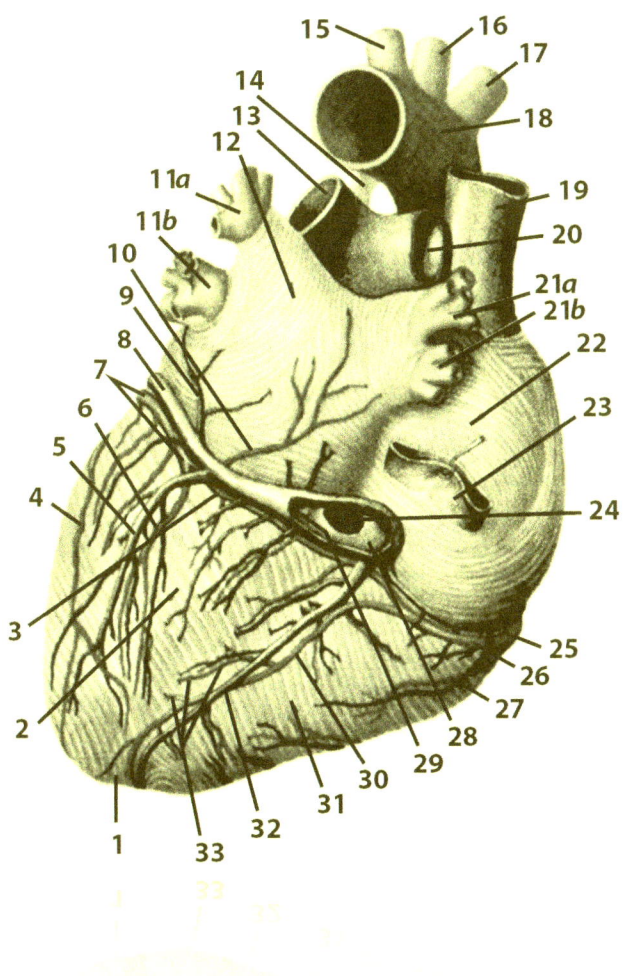

23 – inferior hollow vein 549 671 919 871
24 – opening of coronary sinus 548 641 219 712
25 – small cardiac vein 598 712 918 322
26 – right coronary artery 691 368 519 479
27 – right posterolateral branch 479 691 319 814
28 – valve of the coronary sinus 584 316 219 479
29 – coronary sinus 578 916 219 316
30 – posterior interventricular branch of left coronary artery 589 718 549 641
31 – right cardiac ventricle 598 371 988 011
32 – middle cardiac vein 589 641 298 791
33 – interventricular septal branches 691 314 219 718

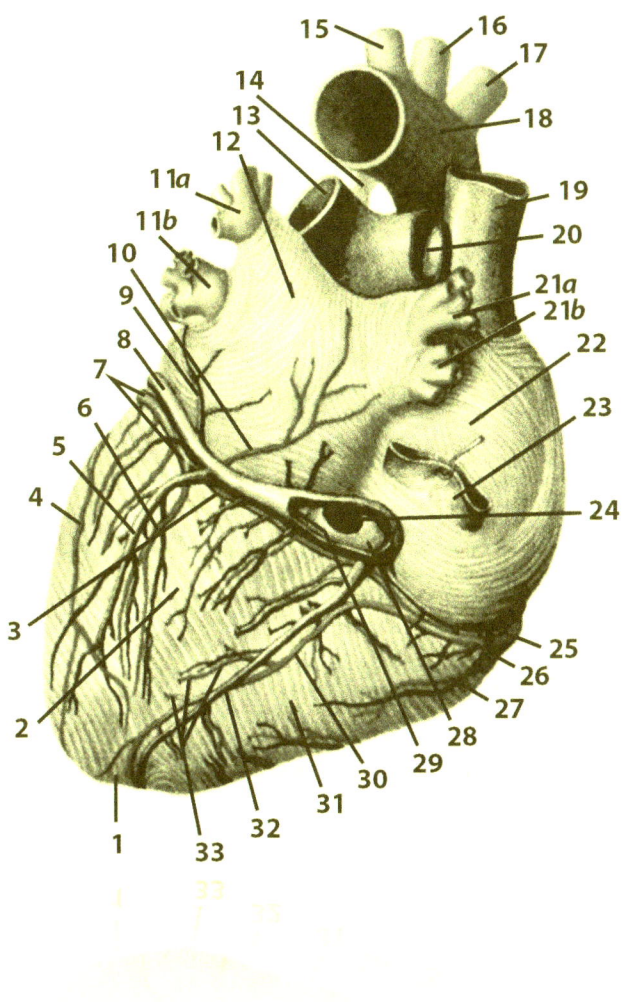

*Fig. 99 Conduction system of the heart 989 808 884 318:*
1 – fleshy trabeculae 194 217 289 678
2 – right cardiac ventricle 598 371 988 011
3 – right peduncle of atrioventricular bundle 319 728 549 641
4 – subendocardial branches of the right ventricle 641 218 514 017
5 – right ventricular papillary muscles 491 318 597 317
6 – tendinous chords of the tricuspid valve 641 318 219 748
7 – right atrioventricular (tricuspid) valve 389 412 819 322
8 – atrioventricular bundle branch block 198 316 398 714
9 – opening of coronary sinus 548 641 219 712
10 – valve of cardiac coronary sinus 584 316 219 479
11 – inferior hollow vein 549 671 919 871
12 – atrioventricular node 169 381 219 714
13 – pectinate muscles 391 689 598 714
14 – oval fossa 394 169 519 718
15 – right atrium 491 016 519 497
16 – interatrial septum 894 158 019 617
17 – sinus node 368 491 298 749
18 – superior hollow vein 398 712 988 012
19 – right superior pulmonary vein 691 894 319 712
20 – openings of pulmonary veins 589 671 298 491
21 – left atrium 518 712 314 887
22 – left superior pulmonary vein (panel) 549 671 298 471
23 – left inferior pulmonary vein 598 649 219 714
24 – opening of the inferior left pulmonary vein 498 712 219 714

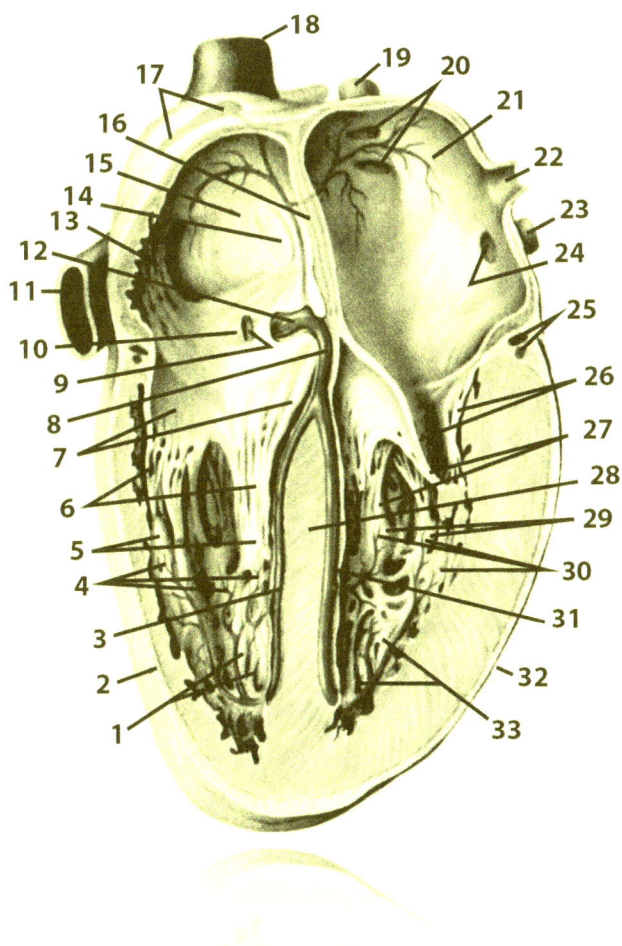

© Грабовой Г.П. 2002

25 – vessels of the heart 549 648 519 716

26 – left atrioventricular (mitral) valve 598 517 818 617

27 – tendinous chords of the mitral valve 794 814 519 714

28 – interventricular septum 548 581 218 491

29 – papillary muscles of left ventricular 467 219 519 712

30 – subendocardial branches of left ventricular 497 518 584 718

31 – left foot of atrioventricular bundle (bundle branch block) 649 191 218 549

32 – left ventricle 589 348 914 918

33 – fleshy trabeculae of left ventricular 468 791 298 745

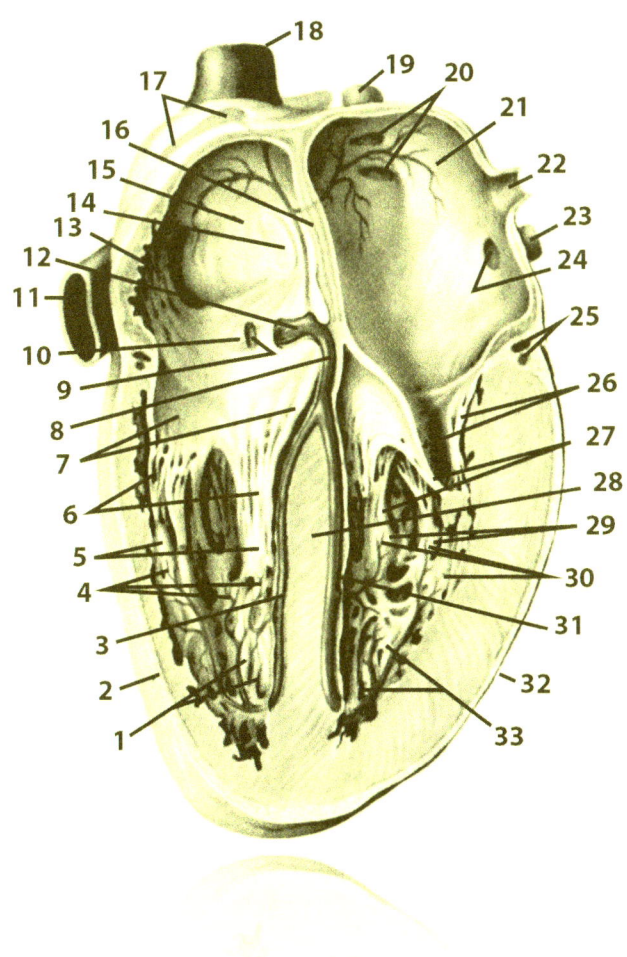

## Veins of the lower extremities 589 712 319 614

*Fig. 100 Veins of the lower extremities 589 712 319 614:*

1 – dorsal venous network of foot 197 298 108 641
2 – dorsal venous arch of foot 194 389 794 216
3 – leg venous network 784 594 316 497
4 – anterior tibial veins 589 714 319 718
5 – knee veins 817 316 368 491
6 – minor subcutaneous foot vein 169 381 379 149
7 – venous network of thigh 497 581 369 794
8 – deep thigh vein 184 517 396 847
9 – lateral veins surrounding the femur bone 649 132 389 714
10 – superficial vein circumflexing iliac bone 317 849 178 471
11 – superficial epigastric vein 491 694 218 713
12 – external iliac vein 999 888 719 898
13 – deep vein circumflexing iliac bone 721 394 549 718
14 – ilio-lumbar veins 548 791 018 216
15 – Lumbar vein 589 712 919 261
16 – inferior hollow vein 549 671 919 871
17 – common iliac vein 548 713 918 781
18 – median sacral vein 598 717 318 917
19 – lateral sacral veins 549 316 298 711
20 – internal iliac vein 549 316 814 787
21 – sacral venous plexus 649 271 298 541
22 – inferior gluteal veins 497 189 369 141

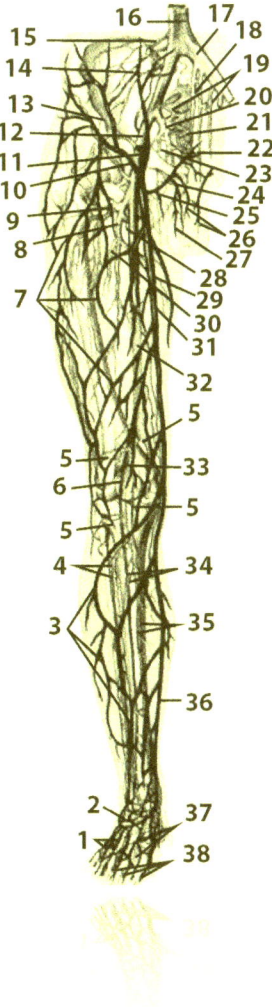

© Грабовой Г.П. 2002

23 – internal pudendal vein 641 894 594 818

24 – vein obturator 318 414 849 161

25 – external pudendal vein 648 143 019 549

26 – superficial dorsal veins of penis 314 647 217 498

27 – anterior scrotal veins 541 314 819 317

28 – dorsal veins surrounding the femur bone 364 981 219 784

29 – accessory saphenous vein 369 489 598 716

30 – perforatory vein 414 548 374 811

31 – great saphenous vein of leg 496 794 894 175

32 – thigh vein 316 584 912 848

33 – vein popliteal 149 721 801 497

34 – peroneal veins 518 364 194 816

35 – posterior tibial veins 479 514 194 817

36 – great saphenous vein of leg 496 794 894 175

37 – dorsal metatarsal veins of foot 648 564 817 219

38 – dorsal digital veins of foot 197 248 594 714

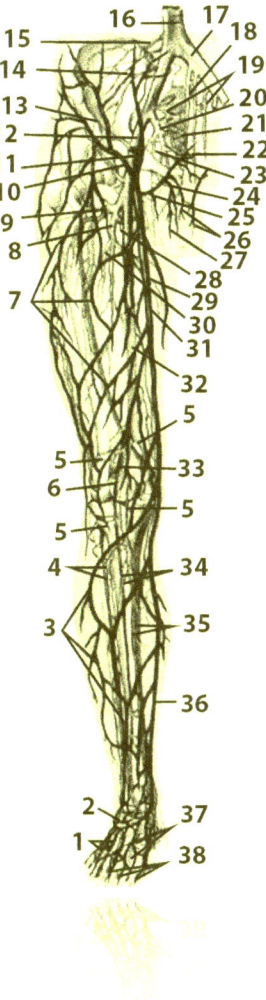

**Arteries, veins and capillaries 219 387 919 887**

*Fig. 101 Microcirculatory channel 549 318 497 561:*

1 – artery 894 547 284 717
2 – arteriole 694 574 895 601
3 – precapillar 608 491 298 491
4 – arteriolo-venular anastomosis 549 316 897 314
5 – precapillar sphincters 649 172 218 371
6 – capillaries 479 821 294 364
7 – capillary sphincters 185 494 016 001
8 – postcapillar 101 498 754 361
9 – venule 669 517 918 394
10 – vein 149 621 818 318

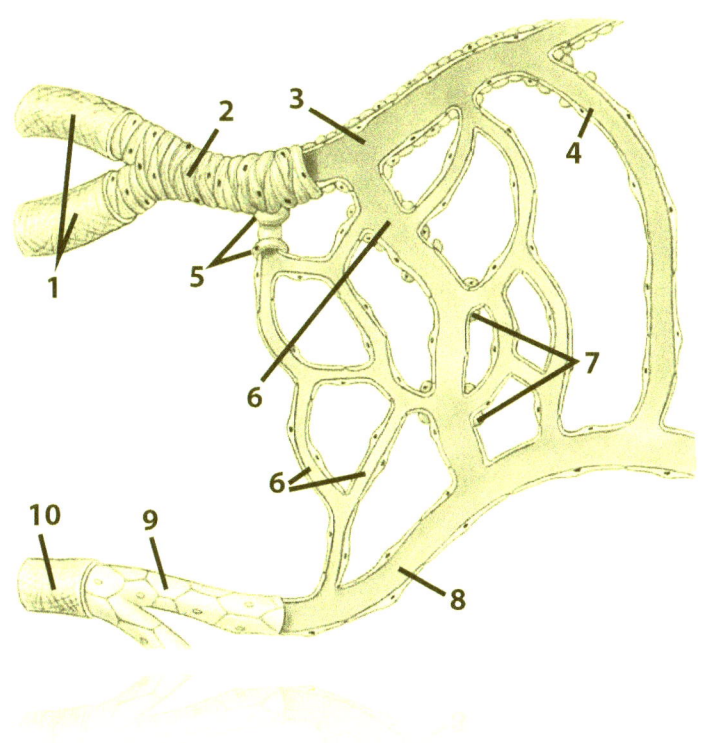

© Грабовой Г.П. 2002

## CENTRAL NERVOUS SYSTEM (CONTINUED) 291 384 074 217

### Brain 814 729 318 818

*Fig. 102 Hypothalamus 918 671 818 971*
*Hypophysis 317 218 219 819:*

1 – oculomotor nerve 519 217 519 217
2 – medial and lateral nuclei of the mastoid body 498 716 219 418
3 – tuber cinereum 898 141 218 718
4 – hypophysis 317 218 219 819
5 – neurohypophysis 814 061 217 041
6 – adenohypophysis (anterior lobe) 518 041 219 498
7 – the core of the funnel (arcuate nucleus) 497 581 264 714
8 – optic nerve 448 817 918 217
9 – supraoptic nucleus 948 516 714 271
10 – inferior medial hypothalamic nucleus 178 491 219 617
11 – pre optical core 718 471 219 648
12 – anterior hypothalamic area 749 164 218 541
13 – dorsomedial hypothalamic nucleus 549 716 218 541
14 – paraventricular nucleus 598 612 317 491
15 – intermediate hypothalamic area 471 218 549 016
16 – posterior hypothalamic nucleus 001 495 018 547
17 – hypothalamic sulcus 016 489 808 489
18 – posterior hypothalamic area 018 418 488 518

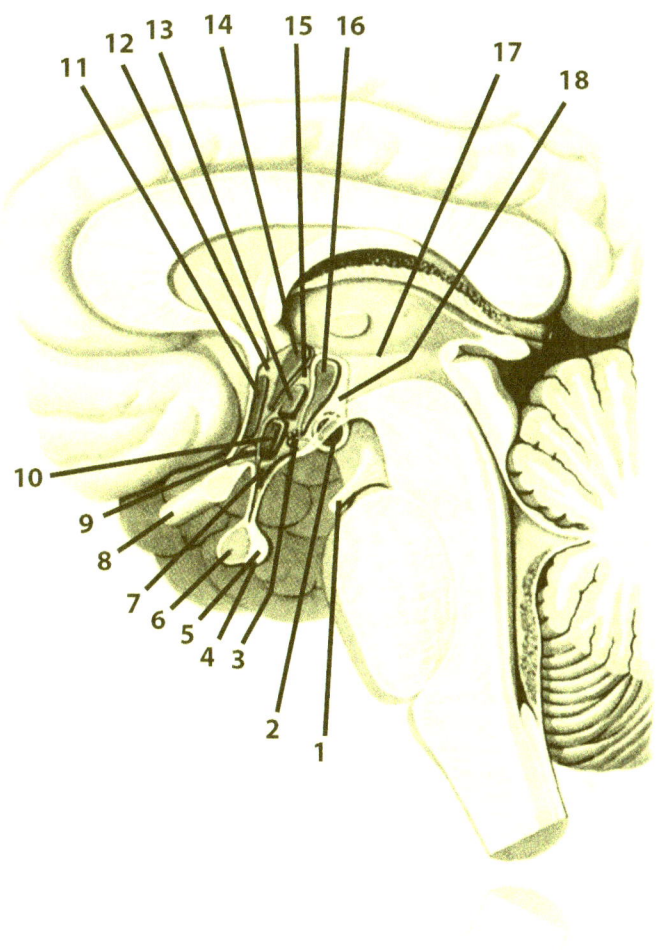

# CONTENTS

**INTRODUCTION** ............................................................................... 4

**HEMOPOIETIC SYSTEM AND IMMUNE PROTECTION SYSTEM 219 648 317 918** ............................... 11

    Central organs of blood formation and immune defense 416 489 319 641 ........................ 14

    Peripheral organs of blood formation and immune defense 794 916 219 481 ..................... 18

    Single of mucous membranes immune system 674 981 219 496 ........................................ 22

**BLOOD CELLS 549681219717** ........................................................ 33

    Leukocytes 694 218 574 271 ............................................ 40

    Agranulocytes 548 274 298 641 ...................................... 40

    Granulocytes 918 547 219 714 ........................................ 44

**DENTOALVEOLAR SYSTEM 216 548 219 716** ............................ 47

    Facial bones of the skull 219 715 819 815 ..................... 47

    Teeth 698 314 819 516 ..................................................... 66

    Organs of oral cavity ...................................................... 126

    Chewing and facial muscles ......................................... 134

    Temporo-mandibular joint ............................................. 138

    Vestibular glands and oral cavity 498 617 219 491 ...... 142

**SPINE** ................................................................................................ 145

**CONNECTIONS, LIGAMENTS AND MUSCLES OF THE SPINE** .. 145

    Spine 214 217 000 819 .................................................... 145

    Vertebrae 498 641 319 048 ............................................. 148

    Spinal motor segment 714 986 219 694 ........................ 169

    Muscles and ligaments of the spine 549 641 894 217 .. 173

Ligaments of the pelvis and hip joint 498 641 798 478 .............................. 184

**MUSCLES AND FASCIA OF**
**BACK AND NECK 798 041 261 509 ........................................................ 189**
**FEMALE PELVIS 494 714 516 841 ........................................................ 200**
    Female external genitalia 519 319 818 678 ................................................ 203
    Internal female sex organs 419 219 808 319................................................ 203

**MAMMARY GLAND 648317219491........................................................ 209**
    The cardiovascular system (continued) 214 700 819 891 .......................... 214
    Arteries and veins of the heart 514 814 219 417.......................................... 242
    Veins of the lower extremities 589 712 319 614 .......................................... 254
    Arteries, veins and capillaries 219 387 919 887 ............................................ 258

**CENTRAL NERVOUS SYSTEM**
**(CONTINUED) 291 384 074 217 ............................................................. 261**
    Brain 814 729 318 818 .................................................................................. 261

Grigori Grabovoi

# Restoration of Matter of Human Being by Concentrating on Number Sequence

# Book 2

www.ingramcontent.com/pod-product-compliance
Lightning Source LLC
Chambersburg PA
CBHW050136240426
43673CB00043B/1694